Emerging Techniques in Aesthetic Plastic Surgery

Guest Editor

LUIZ S. TOLEDO, MD

CLINICS IN PLASTIC SURGERY

www.plasticsurgery.theclinics.com

April 2009 • Volume 36 • Number 2

SAUNDERS an imprint of ELSEVIER, Inc.

W.B. SAUNDERS COMPANY
A Division of Elsevier Inc.

1600 John F. Kennedy Boulevard • Suite 1800 • Philadelphia, Pennsylvania 19103-2899

http://www.theclinics.com

CLINICS IN PLASTIC SURGERY Volume 36, Number 2
April 2009 ISSN 0094-1298, ISBN-13: 978-1-4377-0529-4, ISBN-10: 1-4377-0529-4

Editor: Barbara Cohen-Kligerman

Clinics in Plastic Surgery (ISSN 0094-1298) is published quarterly by Elsevier Inc., 360 Park Avenue South, New York, NY 10010-1710. Months of issue are January, April, July, and October. Business and Editorial Offices: 1600 John F. Kennedy Blvd., Suite 1800, Philadelphia, PA 19103-2899. Periodicals postage paid at New York, NY and additional mailing offices. Subscription prices are $352.00 per year for US individuals, $510.00 per year for US institutions, $177.00 per year for US students and residents, $400.00 per year for Canadian individuals, $596.00 per year for Canadian institutions, $454.00 per year for international individuals, $596.00 per year for international institutions, and $224.00 per year for Canadian and foreign students/residents. To receive student/resident rate, orders must be accompanied by name of affiliated institution, date of term, and the *signature* of program/residency coordinator on institution letterhead. Orders will be billed at individual rate until proof of status is received. Foreign air speed delivery is included in all *Clinics* subscription prices. All prices are subject to change without notice. **POSTMASTER:** Send address changes to *Clinics in Plastic Surgery*, Elsevier Periodicals Customer Service, 11830 Westline Industrial Drive, St. Louis, MO 63146. **Customer Service: 1-800-654-2452 (US). From outside the United States, call 1-314-453-7041. Fax: 1-314-453-5170. E-mail: JournalsCustomerService-usa@elsevier. com (for print support) and JournalsOnlineSupport-usa@elsevier.com (for online support).**

Reprints. For copies of 100 or more of articles in this publication, please contact the Commercial Reprints Department, Elsevier Inc., 360 Park Avenue South, New York, New York 10010-1710. Tel.: (+1) 212-633-3812; Fax: (+1) 212-462-1935; E-mail: reprints@elsevier.com.

Clinics in Plastic Surgery is covered in *Current Contents, EMBASE/Excerpta Medica, Science Citation Index, MEDLINE/ PubMed (Index Medicus), ASCA,* and *ISI/BIOMED.*

Contributors

GUEST EDITOR

LUIZ S. TOLEDO, MD
Chief, Department of Plastic Surgery,
International Modern Hospital, Dubai,
United Arab Emirates

AUTHORS

JUAREZ M. AVELAR, MD
Plastic Surgeon, São Paulo, Brazil

STEPHEN BADYLAK, DVM, MD, PhD
Professor of Surgery, McGowan Institute
for Regenerative Medicine, University of
Pittsburgh, Pittsburgh, Pennsylvania

JAMES BUSH, MBChB, MRCS (Ed)
Renovo Ltd., Manchester, United Kingdom

ROBERT F. CENTENO, MD, MBA
Medical Director, St. Croix Plastic Surgery
and MediSpa, St. Croix, Virgin Islands

DANIEL DEL VECCHIO, MD
Back Bay Plastic Surgery, Boston,
Massachusetts

MICHELLE DE SOUZA, MD
Fellow, The Hunstad Center for Cosmetic
Plastic Surgery, P.A., Charlotte, North Carolina

DANIELLE DUNCAN
Integrative Physiology Student, University
of Colorado, Boulder, Colorado

DIANE DUNCAN, MD, FACS
Private Practice, Ft. Collins, Colorado

JOHN FREUND, BS
McGowan Institute for Regenerative
Medicine, University of Pittsburgh, Pittsburgh,
Pennsylvania

JACK A. FRIEDLAND, MD
Associate Professor of Plastic Surgery, Mayo
Medical School, Rochester, Minnesota; and
Private Practice, Scottsdale, Arizona

ALBERTO GOLDMAN, MD
Clinica Goldman of Plastic Surgery, Porto
Alegre, Brazil

LOREN GOLITZ, MD
Professor, Department of Pathology, University
of Colorado, Denver, Colorado

ROBERT H. GOTKIN, MD, FACS
Cosmetique Dermatology, Laser & Plastic
Surgery, LLP, New York, New York

**DARRYL J. HODGKINSON, MBBS, FRCS (C),
FACS, FACCS**
Director, Cosmetic & Restorative Surgery
Clinic, Double Bay, Sydney, Australia

JOSEPH P. HUNSTAD, MD, FACS
President, The Hunstad Center for Cosmetic
Plastic Surgery, P.A., Charlotte, North Carolina

LYNNE KESEL, DVM
Clinical Veterinarian, Laboratory Animal
Resources, Colorado State University,
Ft. Collins, Colorado

ROGER KHOURI, MD
Dermatology and Plastic Surgery, Key
Biscayne, Florida

ALAN MATARASSO, MD, FACS
Clinical Professor, Department of Plastic
and Reconstructive Surgery, Albert Einstein
College of Medicine; Department of Plastic
Surgery, Manhattan Eye, Ear and Throat
Hospital; Division of Plastic Surgery, Lenox Hill
Hospital; and Private Practice, New York,
New York

RODRIGO NEIRA, MD
Plastic Surgeon, Alberta, Canada

SHARON O'KANE, PhD
Renovo Ltd., Manchester, United Kingdom

TRACY M. PFEIFER, MD, FACS
Department of Plastic Surgery, Manhattan Eye,
Ear and Throat Hospital; Division of Plastic
Surgery, Lenox Hill Hospital; and Private
Practice, New York, New York

PATRÍCIA GUEDES RITTES, MD
Graduate and Post-Graduate in Dermatology,
São Paulo, Brazil

J. PETER RUBIN, MD
Associate Professor of Plastic Surgery,
McGowan Institute for Regenerative Medicine,
University of Pittsburgh, Pittsburgh,
Pennsylvania

GEORGII SULAMANIDZE, MD
Chief, Limited Liability Company APTOS,
Tbilisi, Georgia

MARLEN SULAMANIDZE, MD
Head, Department of Plastic and
Reconstructive Surgery of Central Hospital,
3rd Administration of the Russian Federation
Health Ministry; and Limited Liability Company
APTOS, Tbilisi, Georgia

LUIZ S. TOLEDO, MD
Chief, Department of Plastic Surgery,
International Modern Hospital, Dubai, United
Arab Emirates

V. LEROY YOUNG, MD
BodyAesthetic Plastic Surgery and Skincare
Center, St. Louis, Missouri

Contents

injection lipolysis, many unsuitable patients were treated with this modality. To better understand the way injection lipolysis works, the inclusion and exclusion criteria for patients desiring treatment, and an accurate clinical evaluation format for potential treatment regions, a series of scientific studies was performed in 2007 and early 2008. These studies included a serial histopathology evaluation of treated patients over time, a stem cell study performed with the McGowan Research Institute in Pittsburgh, an animal study performed in conjunction with the Colorado State University veterinary school, and a prospective multicenter clinical trial using injection lipolysis in the back roll region. The purpose of these studies was to determine the way injection lipolysis works, how modifications of the formula and technique change the outcome, the role of each constituent component of various formulas, and the degree of fat reduction and skin retraction that is attainable with these treatments. The influence of depth of injection, distance between injection points, volume of injection, and ratios of constituent components was studied. The degree of topographic contour correction and the amount of volume reduction were evaluated. Following a review of these recent studies, an updated recommendation for the clinical practice of injection lipolysis was formulated.

Comment on "Refinement of Technique in Injection Lipolysis Based on Scientific Studies and Clinical Evaluation"

Juarez M. Avelar

In their article Duncan and colleagues describe scientifically the efficiency of the use of phosphatidylcholine and sodium deoxycholate, which produce adipose lysis to treat small areas of superficial localized adiposities. Previous publications showed the efficiency of this method for correction of localized fat deposits. The authors present a very interesting article with excellent illustrations that is an outstanding contribution to body contour remodeling operations. Such procedures are well indicated to reduce areas of localized adiposities and also to correct remaining local adiposities or irregularities after liposuction.

The Lipodissolve Technique: Clinical Experience

Patrícia Guedes Rittes

This article describes the author's experience with lipodissolve, a nonsurgical treatment to reduce fat deposits via the injection of a single component, phosphatidylcholine, a natural product found in the body. Lipodissolve is a relatively new aesthetic procedure used to dissolve smallish, localized, and defined zones of fat in the face and body.

Review of "The Lipodissolve Technique: Clinical Experience"

Joseph P. Hunstad and Michelle De Souza

Lipodissolve is a relatively new technique of injection lipolysis. Localized areas of fat are treated with the injection of a combination of phosphatidylcholine and deoxycholate. These agents work in concert to reduce fat deposits. The article reviews the results for patients treated with Lipodissolve and other injection lipolysis treatments by Dr. Patricia Rittes, the authors, and other practitioners and researchers. They conclude that properly performed, single-stage surgery that allows the surgeon to address all anatomic levels is preferable to Lipodissolve, pending the results of current and future studies and randomized controlled trials.

Surgisis

Tissue engineering in aesthetic and reconstructive plastic surgery remains an elusive goal. The advent of Surgisis extracellular collagen matrix and its performance characteristics suggest that the use of a bioengineered tissue substitute can meet some of our reconstructive requirements. Incorporation and replacement by host tissue with minimal allergic or immune response seems to be achievable today. The ability to engineer the device, the ready availability of substrate, and its cost effectiveness support the use of Surgisis in aesthetic and reconstructive plastic surgery applications. Future product innovations and engineering seem promising. The permanent role of Surgisis in aesthetic and reconstructive plastic surgery will be determined by its documented long-term performance.

Smartlipo (Laser-Assisted Liposuction)

In the United States, as in many other countries, liposuction is the most commonly performed cosmetic surgical procedure. Advances in technology have enabled surgeons to improve the safety and efficacy of the procedure. One such technological advance is laser-assisted liposuction. This minimally invasive technique employs laser energy in direct contact with adipose tissue to induce lipolysis and, at the same time, coagulate tiny blood vessels and stimulate dermal and subdermal neocollagenesis. These features of laser lipolysis permit a fast, comfortable postoperative recovery, a rapid return to activities of daily living, and excellent skin redraping as a result of laser-induced skin tightening.

This article deals with laser-assisted liposuction. In a question and answer format, it covers such topics as postoperative recovery, skin redraping, and side effects, including its effect on the inflammatory process and on scar and fibrotic tissue and the risk for skin necrosis.

Clinics in Plastic Surgery

FORTHCOMING ISSUES

July 2009

Aesthetic Facial Reconstruction
Stefan O.P. Hofer, MD, PhD, *Guest Editor*

October 2009

Burns
Robert Cartotto, MD, FACS, *Guest Editor*

January 2010

Cutaneous Melanoma
William Dzwierzynski, MD, FACS, *Guest Editor*

RECENT ISSUES

January 2009

Breast Augmentation
Scott L. Spear, MD, FACS, *Guest Editor*

October 2008

Facelifts, Part II
Malcolm D. Paul, MD, FACS, *Guest Editor*

July 2008

Facelifts, Part I
Malcolm D. Paul, MD, FACS, *Guest Editor*

ISSUES OF RELATED INTEREST

Dermatologic Clinics July 2008 (Vol. 26, No. 3)
Spa Dermatology
Neil S. Sadick, MD, *Guest Editor*
Available at http://www.derm.theclinics.com

Oral and Maxillofacial Surgery Clinics of North America February 2009
(Vol. 21, No. 1)
Complications of Cosmetic Facial Surgery
Joseph Niamtu III, DMD, *Guest Editor*
Available at http://www.oralmaxsurgery.theclinics.com

THE CLINICS ARE NOW AVAILABLE ONLINE!

Access your subscription at:
www.theclinics.com

Clinics in Plastic Surgery

Preface

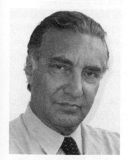

Luiz S. Toledo, MD
Guest Editor

When asked to guest edit an issue of *The Clinics* on emerging techniques, I thought it was important to have a strong American presence, but also to bring techniques that are used internationally but are still not popular in the United States. I looked for surgeons who are on the front line and who conduct research locally and as part of national studies.

Dr. Leroy Young serves on numerous committees of the American Society for Aesthetic Plastic Surgery and the Aesthetic Surgery Education and Research Foundation, and conducts clinical trials at his BodyAesthetic plastic surgery clinic in Saint Louis, Missouri. Dr. Young agreed to write about Juvista, a new product to combat keloid formation, and gave us the name of his associate (at the time) Dr. Robert Centeno, to write about Surgisis, a new injectable tissue filler for the face.

Mesotherapy was developed by the French physician Dr. Michel Pistor in 1952. The technique is so popular today that it has its own board. The members are mostly nonplastic surgeons, because the technique is a minimally invasive procedure to treat various medical conditions with microinjections of conventional or homeopathic medicines, minerals, vitamins, and amino acids. The indications advocated by its users are to eliminate cellulite, treat localized fat, and provide antiaging benefits. This should be of interest to plastic surgeons; however, after more than half a century, it seems that most surgeons have not ever seriously looked into it. We asked Dr. Alan Matarasso, a New York plastic surgeon with an inquisitive mind, who is a prolific author and Clinical Professor of Plastic Surgery at Albert Einstein College of Medicine, to write about his experience with this technique.

Lipodissolve is another technique that is usually confused with mesotherapy. It uses microinjections of two chemicals, phosphatidylcholine and deoxycholate, substances normally secreted and stored in the gall bladder, directly into the subcutaneous fat to remove localized fat deposits over multiple treatment sessions. These chemicals remove the localized fat deposits by emulsifying fat for absorption in the intestine. We invited two of the pioneers of lipodissolve, one from the United States and one from Brazil. From Fort Collins, Colorado, Board-certified plastic surgeon Dr. Diane Duncan is one of the pioneers of the technique in the United States. Dr. Patrícia Rittes from São Paulo, Brazil is a dermatologist who published one of the first clinical works on lipodissolve injections.

The use of lasers in liposuction is not a new idea. It started almost 20 years ago, but the technique is still being perfected. Recently, the use of an internal laser device has become popular, and we asked Dr. Alberto Goldman, a Brazilian plastic surgeon from Porto Alegre who has pioneered the use of laser-assisted liposuction worldwide, to discuss his experience. Dr. Goldman has written an article coauthored by Dr. Robert H. Gotkin, a plastic surgeon from New York. We asked Rodrigo Neira from Cali, Colombia, to peer review the article and he sent the authors a list of questions to stimulate discussion. Drs. Goldman and Gotkin replied to these questions.

One of the areas where research has been particularly important is skin retraction. The heat generated by radiofrequency causes contraction of the collagen fibers and tightens the skin. New collagen forms, and after a few months it produces further delayed tightening. Dr. Darryl Hodgkinson,

Clin Plastic Surg 36 (2009) xi–xii
doi:10.1016/j.cps.2008.12.006

plasticsurgery.theclinics.com

a plastic surgeon from Sydney, Australia, has great clinical experience with the technique. He was one of the first to incorporate this technique in his busy practice and here he shows us his experience.

In 1996, the new minimally invasive technique known as "Russian threading" became very popular, especially among nonplastic surgeons, who liked this simple way to rejuvenate with minimal scarring and short recovery time. The pioneers of the technique were father and son cosmetic surgeons from Tbilisi, Georgia, Drs. Marlen and Georgii Sulamanidze, and they wrote an article on the Aptos thread lift. They use suture threads made with tiny spikes inserted in the subcutaneous tissue at different angles to lift the sagging skin. The barbed-thread lift idea was copied in many countries, with surgeons adding small changes and details, but the idea of a self-supporting thread remained constant.

Dr. Roger Khouri, a plastic surgeon from Miami, Florida, combined two different techniques—tissue expansion and fat grafting—and has been utilizing this to increase breasts without the use of silicone implants, and to reconstruct breasts in a more natural way. He and Dr. Daniel Del Vecchio, a plastic surgeon from Boston, Massachusetts, show their clinical experience with the controversial technique of fat injection in the breasts.

We hope that this issue will bring some science into techniques that are not well known or accepted. Even if we decide not to include these techniques into our practices, they may at least stimulate discussion and make us think of new ways of doing the things we do every day.

On our Web site you will be able to find videos explaining some of the techniques. We hope they can shed more light on these emerging techniques.

When the authors have financial interests in the techniques they present, the article has an appropriate disclaimer.

Finally, I would like to thank the valuable help and guidance of Dr. Robert Goldwyn, a plastic surgery icon with whom I had the pleasure to spend a few days in India and in the Balkans and to discuss the best ways to edit these articles. His vision as the long-standing editor of *Plastic and Reconstructive Surgery Journal* for over 25 years is clear, and in matters where we don't know how to proceed, Bob Goldwyn always has a light, showing the path and avoiding the pitfalls. Thank you for your deep knowledge. Although you were hesitant for me to publish your comments, ethically pointing out that as a retired plastic surgeon it would not be fair to comment on other people's work, I am sure you will recognize here some of your original ideas. You are an inspiration to all of us.

Luiz S. Toledo, MD
PO Box 213522 Jumeirah
Dubai, United Arab Emirates

E-mail address:
ToledoDubai@gmail.com (L.S. Toledo)

Emerging Techniques in Aesthetic Plastic Surgery

Luiz S. Toledo, MD

Why an issue on emerging techniques in aesthetic plastic surgery? Apart from the fact that an issue on old techniques would not be of interest, I do not see any other explanation. As plastic surgeons, we are constantly updating ourselves because science is always evolving and we are always finding new solutions to old problems or, at least, trying to find them. There is always a fine line between the "new" and the experimental and between the breaking news medical advance and quackery. We know that without courageous surgeons who are willing to risk their reputations to breach the frontiers of medical research there would be no progress in medicine (or in any other field for that matter.) So herein we present the work of these doctors. We should analyze their findings and see if there is something that could apply to our practices. Their new techniques might be the solutions for old problems we face every day.

I have always been interested in recent advances in our profession. Since 1989 I have been organizing a meeting called "Recent Advances in Plastic Surgery" (RAPS) to show the most recent techniques in aesthetic surgery. On one hand, it is always good to know what is happening and to be "on the edge." On the other, one must be aware that the new techniques presented have not withstood the test of time; they might work in the long term or they might not. We know that some problems only arise after a few years, such as hypochromia after laser resurfacing that started showing 3 years after the procedure when most surgeons who had bought their lasers had already performed hundreds of procedures.

When invited again to guest edit an issue of *Clinics in Plastic Surgery*, I had no doubt that it should concentrate on new techniques. Maybe some of what is presented herein is not new from the glossy magazines' perspective that demands a new plastic surgery technique every month, but we aim to bring some science into the hubbub about techniques such as mesotherapy and lipodissolve, Russian threads, and "laser lipo," to name a few.

When injections of Lipostabil (phosphatidylcholine) became popular in Brazil a decade ago, every doctor who performed aesthetic medicine and was not a plastic surgeon saw an opportunity to get into the body contour bonanza without having to operate. The media started promoting the new body contour technique without the need for surgery, and every plastic surgeon's office received patients wanting the new injections. At the time I talked to some dermatologists who were friends of mine who were using the medicine imported from Italy. They told me that, although the technique was very painful, it did reduce measurements. When I asked how to prepare the injection I discovered that every formula contained some type of cortisone. Obviously, cortisone works to atrophy fat cells, a well-known fact; however, I found no one using Lipostabil without it, which was one of the reasons I was discouraged from using the technique. The other reason was more of a practical matter, that is, how to control which areas would be affected by the drug. Soon after that, the drug was forbidden in Brazil by Anvisa, the local counterpart of the US Food and Drug Administration (FDA), for lack of scientific data. Nonetheless, one of the pioneers of the technique is a Brazilian dermatologist from São Paulo, Dr. Patricia Rittes, who we invited to write an article for this issue. Dr. Joseph Hunstad, a plastic surgeon in Charlotte, North Carolina, who has experience with lipodissolve writes a comment on Dr. Rittes' article, together with his fellow Dr. Michelle De Souza.

There is a fine line between lipodissolve and mesotherapy. The difference lies mostly in the drugs that are injected and in the depth of

PO Box 213522, Jumeirah, Dubai, United Arab Emirates
E-mail address: toledodubai@gmail.com

Clin Plastic Surg 36 (2009) 177–180
doi:10.1016/j.cps.2008.11.004

injection; however, the principle of dissolving fat through local injections remains the same. To clarify mesotherapy we asked New York plastic surgeon Dr. Alan Matarasso to write an article about his experience with the technique. To date, I have seen few published articles that treat the subject seriously, and if plastic surgeons are going to look into these techniques, there is no one who can guide us better than a physician who has been teaching courses in ASPS congresses for the past decade. I asked Dr. Jack Friedland, a plastic surgeon from Phoenix, Arizona, to comment on Dr. Matarasso's article.

I have had a long experience with using external ultrasound to reduce fat deposits. The machine promises a reduction in measurements and skin retraction; however, my results with the technique were not consistent, because it was difficult to control the power to be applied to each area and obtain the same result. Apart from the power there were many other variables, such as the duration of the application, the area to be treated, the thickness of the skin and fat layer, the drugs mixed into the infiltration solution, the amount of infiltration, and others. Usually what I would see in the postoperative period was a reduction of the measurements in the area without a significant change in its shape. After a few weeks the measurements returned to the original size. I then started combining the external ultrasound application with liposuction to make sure the result was predictable. After a while I abandoned the intraoperative use of the external ultrasound, although I still use it in a weaker mode for postoperative treatments. The same concerns that I faced with the use of external ultrasound I face now with several of the new nonsurgical or minimally invasive techniques.

In the January 2006 issue on lipoplasty, we published an article on the use of the external laser combined with liposuction by Dr. Rodrigo Neira from Cali, Colombia. Dr. Neira performed extensive microscopic studies showing the best potency for the laser machine and the time of application. In the last few years the SmartLipo machine has been developed, a 1064-nm Nd:YAG laser that is introduced in the fat deposit through a 1-mm gauge cannula and that delivers energy directly to the subcutaneous fat cells, causing their rupture. Dr. Alberto Goldman, a Brazilian plastic surgeon from Porto Alegre, has pioneered the use of laser-assisted liposuction and has written an article coauthored by Dr. Robert H. Gotkin, a plastic surgeon from New York. The technique is promoted as less invasive than conventional liposuction. The theory is to destroy fat cells and coagulate tissue to obtain tighter skin on the face

and body. The emitted energy should also induce collagen retraction and tissue tightening. Because the laser coagulates small blood vessels, there should be less bleeding, swelling, and bruising than with conventional liposuction, and faster healing and recovery.

I started using this machine over a year ago and have had mixed results. My experience usually does not match that of the authorities who promote its use. In some of my cases I have had skin laxity, bleeding, seromas, and delayed healing. I must admit I rarely used the SmartLipo alone without suctioning the melted fat. In some of my cases the expected skin retraction did not happen, and, when it happened, the result took at least 2 months to show. My impression of this machine so far is that it is a good marketing tool. Patients are attracted by the word "laser." It projects an image of an advanced surgeon who uses contemporary techniques of medicine. An ethical problem arises, that is, the question of whether I am misleading my patients. I believe the answer is no. Many surgeons have had extremely successful experiences with the SmartLipo machine, and I am doing exactly what I have learned from them. We asked Dr. Neira to peer review the article, and he sent the author, Dr. Goldman, a list of questions to stimulate discussion to which he replied.

How many times have we performed a facelift and, after 6 months, looked at the patient and wished we had pulled the skin a little more because the result was not as tight as it should be. We know it would be unwise to have pulled more during the surgery due to the risk of skin necrosis, and that it is too soon to suggest a revision at such short follow-up. Nevertheless, we wish there was something we could do to improve the skin tone. A new array of noninvasive treatments is being developed for this problem, ranging from fractional laser to radiofrequency treatment. In this issue Dr. Darryl Hodgkinson, a plastic surgeon from Sydney, Australia, looks into the use of radiofrequency applied with the Thermage machine, which promises skin retraction and rejuvenation with the formation of new collagen. Whenever a new treatment promises to cure cellulite or stretch marks (striae), a red light starts flashing in my brain. These problems are two of the most common aesthetic issues, and we still have no efficient treatment for them. It is no surprise that much research is ongoing in these two areas; however, to date, the results have been disappointing. We can certainly improve the appearance of cellulite areas with a combination of liposuction, dissection, and fat injection, but we are not treating the cause of the problem, and, sooner or later, the irregularities tend to reappear.

The same goes for stretch marks. We can sometimes cut off the affected skin, such as in the lower abdomen, leaving a scar in its place; however, once the dermis is ruptured and the skin has lost its power to retract, the damage is irreversible. Other treatments prescribed include microdermabrasion, chemical peels, and laser resurfacing. In the article on this problem we see some impressive abdominal and arm skin retraction with radiofrequency. Although the results seem good in the photographs, we need to know more to be able to draw a conclusion about the efficiency of radiofrequency in cosmetic surgery. Dr. Hodgkinson's article reveals his clinical impressions 6 months post treatment. He states, "Numerous patients have returned after 6 months as they are impressed by the result, and have second treatments. The skin complexion seems to be improved."

In 1985 we performed fat grafting in great quantities in São Paulo to correct facial atrophy, augment buttocks and calves, and even breasts, and have continued doing so for the last 2 decades. We first presented our 18-month follow-up of fat grafting at the International Society of Aesthetic Plastic Surgery Congress in New York in 1987 together with Dr. Paulo Matsudo, a plastic surgeon from São Paulo. The *Aesthetic Plastic Surgery Journal* published our "Experience with Injected Fat Grafting"[1] in 1988. In that article we presented 33 cases of fat injection in the breasts. Our results were good, but in 1987 there was a discussion in the *Plastic and Reconstructive Surgery Journal* about the possibility of confusion with breast tumors and the fat graft calcification. In 1987 we stopped fat injections of the breasts because our diagnostic equipment was not capable of differentiating between the two types of calcification. In 2007 the American Society of Plastic Surgery (ASPS) held a panel presenting the "new wave" of doctors who were now injecting fat in the breasts. The panel also presented radiologists who showed new equipment now able to precisely diagnose the fat grafting calcification. At the end of the panel when asked if they were finally endorsing fat injection to the breast as a safe technique, the panel members replied yes. This policy will have to be reinforced by the ASPS, because there was not much time for discussion or questions. I believe the answer is in having the right equipment. We invited Dr. Roger Khouri from Miami to show us his experience with fat injection after vacuum expansion of the breasts. He presents this technique together with

Dr. Daniel Del Vecchio from Boston. One of the serious technical problems when performing fat injection is how to inject under a scar or a retracted area. The fat cells seem to go everywhere but into the area that needs filling. Dr. Khouri has solved this problem by using a vacuum pump like a tissue expander before the fat injection, preparing that area to accept the graft. The system is not new; it has been used for decades for penis and breast enlargement. Dr. Khouri has perfected the device, and with its use he can treat not only small breasts but also postmastectomy areas, preparing the retracted tissue for enlargement with autologous fat.

For several reasons we did not include a discussion of stem cell research in this issue. In the January 2006 issue on liposuction, the basic science aspects of the subject were covered. Further discussion would be warranted if published clinical data on adipose stem cells could be presented; however, to date, serious clinical data are still not available. Obviously, the media hype on stem cells is widely used by many doctors who claim to be doing stem cell injections. To some extent this is true, because if one injects fat, consequently one injects stem cells with it; however, this injection is not yet done with the level of purity we believe stem cell research will be able to produce in the near future.

The Baker phenol formula from 1963 has dominated the peel market for decades. This phenol peel has been used successfully for over 40 years for deep chemical peeling and produces reliable results. It is a serious procedure that must be performed under strict surveillance by an anesthesiologist. The patient should be watched carefully for signs of toxicity. It has precise indications and is especially good for deep perioral wrinkles, periorbital wrinkles and crow's feet, forehead lines, and other severe wrinkles.

In 2000 Dr. Gregory Hetter, a plastic surgeon from Las Vegas, Nevada, demonstrated prizewinning work on the effect of the croton oil peel. Since then many new formulas have been launched under different names and different solutions. I watched a presentation of the Timepeel solution by Dr. Sae-hyun Pyun at the European Masters in Anti-aging & Aesthetic Medicine Congress in Paris in 2007 and was very impressed by the results. I used the Baker formula in the 1970s, trichloroacetic acid (TCA) peels in the 1980s, alpha hydroxy acid peels in the 1990s, and had a brief exposure to the Exoderm formula in my clinic. Since I have moved to Dubai my patient population has changed. I see more dark-skinned patients here than in Brazil, and if there is something I do not want to have, it is a complication on a local patient.

I started using Russian threads in São Paulo in 1997. Imported from Russia, the threads were dark blue with very fine spikes. The thread was in many cases not long enough and too thin to support some areas, and the dark color would sometimes show under the skin of very fair-skinned patients. As is true for everything in plastic surgery, a Brazilian company started making a longer, transparent polypropylene thread with thicker double-helix spikes. The price was one quarter that of the Russian thread. There was a big media campaign, and many patients wanted the new technique. It was a simple procedure performed under local anesthesia with little downtime. The subjective results were very good. Many times I would not see much difference between a before and after picture, but patients simply loved the result, continued coming back for more, and sent their friends. Patients liked the immediate lift obtained by the thread and did not mind if they had to return for revisions. In 2004 I organized an RAPS meeting in Belgrade together with Dr. Mico Djuricic and brought specialists from Brazil to perform live surgery and demonstrate the technique. As we do every year, the 1-year postoperative results were shown at the next congress, and it was disappointing to see that most results had disappeared after 6 months. When I asked a cosmetic surgeon from Georgia, Dr. Marlen Sulamanidze, the inventor of the Russian thread, and his son Georgi to write about their experience with the Aptos thread, I wanted to have the experts' opinion for the first time in a plastic surgery publication. They wrote an excellent article clarifying many obscure points in the technique.

We could not have an issue on emerging techniques without some clinical articles on new substances. Dr. Leroy Young from St. Louis, Missouri, with Drs. James Bush and Sharon O'Kane, present new ways to improve or minimize scarring using avotermin (TGFβ3), a new class of prophylactic medicines that may promote the regeneration of normal skin and improve scar appearance, showing significant improvements when compared with placebo and resulting in less noticeable scars that more closely resemble the surrounding skin.

From St. Croix in the Caribbean, Dr. Robert Centeno writes an article on Surgisis Acellular Collagen Matrix, a porcine intestinal mucosa–derived product made commercially available in 1998 after FDA 510K clearance for soft tissue reconstruction. Application of this device in plastic surgery applications has been recent. We are now at a stage when a bioengineered tissue substitute can meet some of the reconstructive requirements in plastic surgery.

REFERENCE

1. Matsudo PK, Toledo LS. Experience with injected fat grafting. Aesthetic Plast Surg 1988;12:35–8.

Mesotherapy and Injection Lipolysis

Alan Matarasso, MD, FACS[a,b,c,d,*], Tracy M. Pfeifer, MD, FACS[b,c,e]

KEYWORDS

- Mesotherapy • Subcutaneous fat reduction
- Injection lipolysis • Phosphatidylcholine
- Sodium deoxycholate

Plastic surgeons continue to seek refinement, improvements, and safety in existing techniques, and patients often seek less-invasive procedures, improved results and solutions for complex problems.

These are some of the reasons that mesotherapy and injection lipolysis have experienced some popularity in the United States. Although some studies are emerging in the English medical literature to document the safety and efficacy of injection lipolysis, in the United States the enthusiasm among patients and physicians largely has been driven by reports in the lay press and the quest for permanent fat reduction by nonsurgical methods. Because of this and for other reasons, controversy has surrounded mesotherapy and injection lipolysis. The primary concern is that the clinical application of these methods in patients has preceded rigorous scientific study of these agents and their application that would be necessary to establish safety and efficacy required for US Food and Drug Administration (FDA) approval.

The purpose of the first part of this article is to familiarize the reader with the evolution of mesotherapy, injection lipolysis, and the use of phosphatidylcholine and deoxycholate for subcutaneous fat reduction. There is an emphasis on the underlying basic science of fat metabolism and the biochemistry of phosphatidylcholine, so that practitioners will be able to understand future published research on these topics. The second half of the article details some personal experience with injection lipolysis.

MESOTHERAPY

Recently, there has been a renewed interest in the technique of mesotherapy as a method of reducing subcutaneous fat for body contouring. Most sources credit Pistor with having developed the technique of mesotherapy in France in 1952.[1] Practitioners of mesotherapy in France, however, can trace the roots of mesotherapy to 2000 BC in China (T Pfeifer and DI Duncan, personal communication, 2008). Others place the time even earlier at 3000 BC. The modern era of mesotherapy, however, began in approximately 1952, when Pistor injected a partially deaf patient with intravenous procaine for the treatment of an acute asthma attack.[2] This was a standard treatment for asthma at the time. Surprisingly, the patient experienced improved hearing for several hours. Noting the temporarily improved hearing after intravenous procaine injection, Pistor began injected procaine into the superficial dermis in close proximity to the ear. Surprisingly, in some patients a reduction in cervical pain was noted. According to Petit, a mesotherapy practitioner in France, Pistor was marginalized and seen as a healer rather than as a physician. Pistor subsequently coined the term mesotherapy to describe treatment of the mesoderm. He believed that the local injections had an effect on tissues originating from the mesoderm, one of the three primary germ layers of the embryo, which develops into the dermis of the skin, connective tissue, muscle, and the circulatory system. At its inception, mesotherapy referred

a Department of Plastic and Reconstructive Surgery, Albert Einstein College of Medicine, New York, NY, USA
b Department of Plastic Surgery, Manhattan Eye, Ear and Throat Hospital, New York, NY, USA
c Division of Plastic Surgery, Lenox Hill Hospital, New York, NY, USA
d Private Practice, 1009 Park Avenue, New York, NY 10028, USA
e Private Practice, 565 Park Avenue, New York, NY 10028, USA
* Corresponding author.
E-mail address: matarasso@aol.com (A. Matarasso).

Clin Plastic Surg 36 (2009) 181–192
doi:10.1016/j.cps.2008.11.002
0094-1298/08/$ – see front matter © 2009 Published by Elsevier Inc.

specifically to intradermal injections, and most publications still define mesotherapy as intracutaneous injections. Mesotherapy, however, has evolved to include injections into the epidermis and dermis, subcutaneous injections and regional injections. The French Society of Mesotherapy was founded in 1964, and the applications of mesotherapy soon expanded. In 1980, the Cercles d'Etude et de Recherche en Mésothérapie (CERM) was formed. The CERM is a research group formed to study mesotherapy. In 1982, Pistor created the International Society of Mesotherapy. In 1987, mesotherapy was recognized by the French Academy of Medicine as a medical specialty. Also in 1987, the first advanced degree in mesotherapy was established in Marseille, and in 1996, Petit organized a degree program in Bordeaux. Over the years, mesotherapy has gained acceptance in many countries, and in France, both physicians and patients recognize it as an integral part of health care.

The goal of mesotherapy injections is to stimulate the mesoderm for various biological purposes. The substances injected include: vasodilators, anti-inflammatory medication, muscle relaxants, proteolytic enzymes, vitamins, minerals, plant extracts, vaccines, antibiotics, hormones, hormone blockers, and anesthetics.[3] Recently, phosphatidylcholine and deoxycholate have been used in subcutaneous injections. Most mesotherapy formulas contain a vasodilator. The reason for this is not entirely clear, but recent work by Duncan has shown that the vasodilator results in a more rapid clearing or uptake of injected phosphatidylcholine and deoxycholate (TM Pfeifer, and DI Duncan, personal communication, 2008). Thus, the vasodilator may be useful for patients who have conditions requiring vasodilation for treatment or those in whom systemic uptake of the injected medication is desirable. Generally, the formula or cocktail injected is determined by the practitioner, according to the needs of the particular patient. Thus, standardized formulas for the most part do not exist. The lack of standard ingredients and formulas further contributes to the inability to extrapolate data and compare results. Mesotherapy has been advocated for treating an assortment of conditions as varied as chronic pain, vascular disease, psoriasis, and rheumatoid arthritis. In France, mesotherapy primarily is used to treat nonaesthetic conditions including sports injuries and chronic pain; its use for aesthetic purposes is limited. In the United States, practitioners primarily have used mesotherapy for aesthetic purposes including: the treatment of cellulite, weight loss, spot weight loss, skin rejuvenation, hair loss, and the treatment of facial rhytids. The theory is that mesotherapy helps reverse the physiology of the condition. The compounds injected are usually a combination of different ingredients and are chosen based on the pathophysiology of the disease. For example, rheumatoid arthritis is treated using anti-inflammatory medications and plant agents thought to control inflammation.

In the United States, the first reports of mesotherapy appeared in the lay press in December 2001.[4] In January 2003, *People* magazine reported that the singer Roberta Flack lost 30 pounds on a weight loss program that included mesotherapy administered by a physician who studied mesotherapy in Paris; the story also reported that mesotherapy treatments to the face resulted in "a youthful glow."[5] After these initial reports, mesotherapy received a significant amount of press coverage in the United States. Patients began requesting mesotherapy and very little, if any, scientific information written in English was available to American physicians. At the time, most of the published medical literature was in French. Jacque Le Coz, former president of the French Society of Mesotherapy, has written extensively on the subject of mesotherapy.[6] Although all of his books are written in French, in 2008 he translated his most recent book into English.[7] Recently, Madhère of New York edited a textbook on mesotherapy published in English. The book provides an overview on the topic and specific information on mesotherapy not readily available to American physicians.[8] The book includes chapters written by widely respected French practitioners of mesotherapy and American leaders in the field of mesotherapy.

Multiple injection techniques exist for mesotherapy, and there is debate within the community of mesotherapy practitioners as to which techniques are most appropriate. Injections can be:

Intraepidermic (IED)
Papule (IDS), in which a bleb is raised at the junction of epidermis with the dermis
Nappage, in which two to four injections are made per second, spaced 2 to 4 mm apart at an angle of 30° to 60°
Point-by-point (PPP) injections are placed in the dermis at approximately 4 mm depth
Specific systemic mesotherapy injections are placed in the deep dermis and hypodermis for treating rheumatologic disorders and pain management
Mesoperfusion injections involve the slow injection over 30 to 90 minutes of 2.5 to 10 cc, placed 4 to 13 mm deep, for treating insomnia and chronic pain

Subcutaneous injections, which are being used in the treatment of subcutaneous fat, as in injection lipolysis

Mesotherapy can involve 8 to 300 injections per treatment; treatments are weekly or every other week. The number of treatments varies and ranges between 3 and 15 injection sessions, depending on the condition. Injections are administered either by a standard syringe, usually either 5 or 10 cc, or using a hand-held device, called a mesogun, which has a syringe and needle (27 or 30g) attached; the volume of injection can be varied. Injection needles are typically 4 mm long. The volume of injection is usually very small. Mesoguns may be either automatic or semiautomatic, and they can be purchased for approximately $2000 to $8000.[9] Fully automatic mesoguns advance the needle and deliver the injection. Semiautomatic mesoguns require manual advancement of the needle or trigger-operated delivery of the injection. One mesogun is approved by the FDA, the Dermotherap by USA Meso.

In the United States, the clinical application of mesotherapy in patients is controversial for several reasons. The primary criticism of mesotherapy is that it is unproven from a scientific standpoint. The lack of standardized formulas and protocols makes it virtually impossible to validate results and reports of efficacy by replication of studies. Widely practiced in Europe and South America, the bulk of specific reports on mesotherapy are published in French, Italian, and Spanish literature.[10–18] There is a paucity of rigorous scientific studies published in the English medical literature regarding the safety and efficacy of mesotherapy.[19] The overall safety of mesotherapy is not well-documented. There are reports in the literature, however, of complications and side effects including ulceration, prolonged swelling, pain, panniculitis, skin ulceration, abscess, hematoma, psoriasis, atypical mycobacterial infections, urticaria, and hyperpigmentation.[20–31]

A second criticism is that although some of the individual ingredients injected during mesotherapy are known, these substances usually are used in combination. The individual practitioner often determines the particular combination of ingredients used for a given treatment. There is concern about unknown interactions between the medications combined in each cocktail. Furthermore, the 'Tratado de Mesotherapia' is a handbook only published in Spanish, describing the various applications of mesotherapy, active agents used, and recommended protocols; it includes an extensive bibliography.[32] It is available through Laboratories Mesoestetic Limited, a company based in Spain

that also manufactures and sells the products used mesotherapy.[33] At this time, an English translation is not available. One publication in the English medical literature describes the practitioner's protocols for reduction of subcutaneous fat, treatment of cellulite, mesoglow (skin rejuvenation), and mesohair (treatment of hair loss).[19] Although the exact formulas used are given, a precise description of injection protocol is not provided.

As in any other aspect of medicine, physicians interested in practicing mesotherapy need training in its methods. This includes knowing the exact medications used, understanding the pharmacology of medications used in mesotherapy, technical training on appropriate delivery methods, and understanding the possible complications and contraindications of the procedure. In some instances, physicians can access this information only through courses for which there is a fee to the physician participant. This commercialization of the sharing of scientific information that may benefit patients is somewhat in contradiction with the tenets of medicine. This proprietary approach conflicts with the time-honored tradition of an altruistic free and open exchange of scientific information in the interest of providing care and treatment for patients.[34]

Additional controversy arises from the fact that in some countries, including the United States, practitioners of mesotherapy include both properly trained medical personnel and unlicensed practitioners. Brazil banned the use of Lipostabil in mesotherapy in part because of its use by unlicensed practitioners and resulting complications.[35] In the United States, many medispas offer mesotherapy administered by unsupervised nurses or aestheticians to their clients without having a physician evaluate and treat the patient. In addition, other nonphysician professionals such as chiropractors, dentists, and massage therapists are starting to offer mesotherapy. Nonsurgeon physicians may take a course to learn about mesotherapy. This leads to practitioners of mesotherapy who are not fully trained in the technique. Additionally, these practitioners do not have the ability to fully evaluate the patient's condition and offer appropriate alternative treatments. Moreover, they may not be able to diagnose and treat a complication. Some states require a physician be on site and have evaluated the patient before treatment; others do not. Even in states requiring on-site supervision and evaluation by physicians, medispas staffed only by nurses or aestheticians continue to offer mesotherapy to their clients.

The practice of mesotherapy by unlicensed personnel has had several unfortunate consequences. First, when complications occur, it is often when mesotherapy is performed by nonmedical personnel. Second, with medispas and salons offering mesotherapy, the public falsely assumes that mesotherapy is a procedure akin to other beauty treatments such as, for example, waxing. Patients assume mesotherapy is not the practice of medicine and therefore harmless. What should be considered a medical treatment thus is trivialized, and the entire technique and treatment modality is harmed. Patients are unaware of the potential complications of mesotherapy, can be victims of unscrupulous practitioners of mesotherapy, and may fall prey to aggressive marketing practices by businesses commercializing mesotherapy for profit. Third, patients know that the practice of medicine is regulated by the state and federal government. Therefore, patients believe that if mesotherapy is a medical treatment and being administered by nonmedical personnel, that the treatment must be safe, because the government allows this practice. Most physicians probably would agree that procedures that can result in deformity and other significant complications should be considered the practice of medicine. What constitutes the practice of medicine, however, is defined by state law, which varies from state to state. Some states consider a procedure that results in penetration of the skin to be the practice of medicine. Other states apparently do not consider mesotherapy to be the practice of medicine. Even in states in which mesotherapy meets the definition of the practice of medicine, enforcement of state laws and statues may be difficult.

The aforementioned issues, including the lack of scientific information, unregulated practice and failure to share information in the usual scientific tradition has led to serious doubt and skepticism about mesotherapy and the appropriateness of physicians offering these nonproven treatments to their patients.

Mesotherapy injection ingredients are inexpensive and easy to acquire. For example, aminophylline 25 mg/mL, 20 cc vial can be purchased for approximately $2.25 per vial.[36] Although the medications used in mesotherapy may be FDA-approved for other indications, no medication is approved by the FDA for use in mesotherapy. It is important to clarify that the FDA does not consider the use of FDA-approved drugs in mesotherapy to be an off-label use. The FDA has three categories for drugs and devices used in people:

1. Approved for a specific use (labeled and approved by the FDA for marketing)
2. Approved and permitted for off-label use
3. Nonapproved (not approved by the FDA for any purpose and ineligible for off-label use)

With a few exceptions such as collagenase, hyaluronidase, local anesthetics, and calcitonin, the medications used in mesotherapy are not approved by the FDA for intradermal or subcutaneous injection.[37] FDA drug approval includes the delivery method. Thus, if one injects a medication intradermally that is FDA approved for intravenous administration, this does not constitute off-label usage. This would be a nonapproved use. Off-label usage refers to the use of an FDA-approved drug, including method of administration, for an indication other than for which it was approved.

MESOTHERAPY FOR SUBCUTANEOUS FAT REDUCTION

Mesotherapy has been used for several years in Europe and South America for body contouring and has been advocated as a nonsurgical alternative to liposuction.

Mesotherapy for fat reduction often is used in conjunction with dietary modification, hormone replacement therapy, exercise, and nutritional supplements. Thus, it can be difficult to precisely identify the contribution of mesotherapy to any reduction in subcutaneous fat, if there is one.

Park recently examined the results of mesotherapy in 20 women enrolled in a prospective, case-controlled study.[38] The study was designed to evaluate the effectiveness of mesotherapy using aminophylline, buflomedil (non-FDA approved vasodilator) and lidocaine to reduce subcutaneous fat in the medial thigh. The change in fat was evaluated by measuring circumference and by CT scanning. The authors found there was no difference in circumference or any difference in cross-sectional area or thickness of the fat layer by CT scan. In contrast, other practitioners report a reduction in subcutaneous fat after mesotherapy. In 1995, Greenway reported a reduction in thigh girth in women injected with isoproterenol.[39] Patients in this study and in a second study by Greenway, who applied topical creams containing aminophylline and other substances, also experienced a reduction in thigh girth.[40]

In 2004, two plastic surgeons presented an abstract evaluating the use of mesotherapy for body contouring and cellulite treatment.[41] Forty patients were enrolled in a double-blinded, prospective study; a single body region was treated by mesotherapy on a weekly basis for 5 weeks, followed by monthly maintenance therapy. The patients were separated into four groups. Group 1 (N=10) received mesotherapy treatments unilaterally; group 2 (N=10) received treatments bilaterally. Group 3 (N=10) received mesotherapy in association with dietary modification and exercise, and group 4 (N=10) received saline placebo injections. Patients were surveyed by questionnaire and evaluated by a physician who was blinded. Objective evaluation included measurement of circumference and pinch test. Most patients treated with mesotherapy reported a noticeable difference in the treated area (groups 1 and 3, 18 out of 20; group 2, 7 out of 10). Circumference measurements decreased in most patients who were treated. The average decrease in circumference was 2.6 cm at the waist and 1.8 cm at the thigh; the greatest circumference decrease was 3.8 cm at the waist and 2.5 cm at the thigh. In all treated groups, the appearance of cellulite was reduced dramatically. No major complications occurred; several minor complications were observed. These included transient erythema of the treated area in six patients, one localized infection at an injection site, minimal ecchymosis in five patients, and significant ecchymosis in one patient.

Research is starting to clarify the mechanisms by which mesotherapy for reduction of subcutaneous fat and cellulite reduction possibly could work. It is known that lipolysis of fat stored in adipocytes is regulated by alpha-2 and beta-adrenoreceptors on the adipocyte cell surface. Beta-receptor activity increases lipolysis, and alpha-2 receptor activity inhibits beta-receptors.

A theoretic possibility is that compounds that promote beta-activation and alpha-2 inhibition may increase rates of lipolysis. In the case of mesotherapy for reduction in subcutaneous fat and cellulite reduction, the theory is that stimulation of the adipocyte beta-adrenergic receptor causes a resultant increase in lipolysis. Isoproterenol, one of the agents commonly used in mesotherapy, is a beta-receptor stimulator. In addition to beta-receptor stimulators, other substances including estrogen and thyroid as well as methylxanthines caffeine and aminophylline are known to increase lipolysis.[42,43] Several publications describe enhanced lipolysis in adipose tissue perfused with isoproterenol.[44,45] In 2007, Caruso reported that isoproterenol, aminophylline, yohimbine, and Melilotus stimulate lipolysis as evaluated by an in vitro assay.[46] Others, however, believe that the increased lipolysis seen after beta-receptor stimulation by mesotherapy injections is fundamentally different from that seen after injection lipolysis with phosphatidylcholine and deoxycholate (DI Duncan and P Rubin, personal communication. When beta-receptor stimulators such as epinephrine are injected, a transient increase is seen in blood triglyceride levels. This might correspond to a temporary decrease in adipocyte triglyceride levels. After the effects of beta-receptor stimulation have worn off, the triglycerides are restored in the adipocyte. Under this hypothesis, one can presume no permanent change in the adipocyte volume. The theory postulates that cell wall disruption and subsequent necrosis of the adipocyte must occur for a permanent reduction in subcutaneous fat to occur. With respect to cellulite, enhanced lipolysis also has been postulated as the mechanism by which cellulite is improved after mesotherapy. One recent study using microdialysis assays, however, showed no difference in rates of lipolysis between cellulite and noncellulite adipose tissue.[47] Other proposed mechanisms for how mesotherapy results in spot fat reduction include enhanced circulation and alterations in connective tissue.

INJECTION LIPOLYSIS WITH PHOSPHATIDYLCHOLINE

As discussed previously, mesotherapy has been applied to the reduction of subcutaneous fat. Recently, there has been interest in injection lipolysis, the subcutaneous injection of phosphatidylcholine and deoxycholate for subcutaneous fat reduction.

Phosphatidylcholine is a naturally occurring glycerolphospholipid composed of glycerol with two fatty acids and choline attached. It has three important functions:

1. It emulsifies dietary fat, thereby playing a vital role in digesting dietary fat.
2. It is a component of the apolipoproteins essential to cholesterol metabolism.
3. It is an essential component of cell membranes.[48]

Phosphatidylcholine contributes to the proper metabolism of fat and cell membrane integrity, is important in neuron conduction, increases the solubility of cholesterol, is the precursor to acetylcholine, and is a surfactant in the alveoli of the lungs. Phosphatidylcholine is able to emulsify blood fats, resulting in increased surface area of chylomicrons, allowing quicker breakdown of triglycerides by the enzyme lipoproteinlipase.

Phosphatidylcholine is consumed in a normal diet and is also available as oral supplements. Oral phosphatidylcholine is considered a dietary supplement and therefore is not regulated by the FDA. Oral phosphatidylcholine supplements are used to guard against low blood choline levels and to restore blood choline levels in patients suffering from select brain disorders.[49] It may have a role for treating Alzheimer's disease.[50] Lecithin, composed of a phosphate group, choline, fatty acids, glycerol, glycolipids, triglycerides, and phospholipids including phosphatidylcholine, phosphatidylethanolamine, and phosphatidylinositol, is a common source of oral phosphatidylcholine. Phosphatidylcholine is also available in an injectable form. Injectable phosphatidylcholine is not approved by the FDA. Phosphatidylcholine, however, is a component of several FDA-approved intravenous drugs.[51] Injectable phosphatidylcholine can be obtained through compounding pharmacies, the Internet, or overseas (Mesoestetic, Limited, Barcelona, Spain).

In the Russian literature in particular, there are many reports on the positive effects of phosphatidylcholine on lipid profiles and cholesterol levels. It has been used oversees to treat liver disease, including hepatitis, cirrhosis, fatty liver, and drug- or toxin-induced liver damage.[52] In the United States, basic science research has shown positive effects of phosphatidylcholine on cholesterol levels, alcohol-induced mitochondrial injury, alcohol-induced hepatocyte apoptosis, and liver fibrosis.[52–56]

In Europe, intravenous phosphatidylcholine, marketed under the brand name Lipostabil, manufactured by Sanofi-Aventis Group (Paris, France). It comes in 5 cc ampoules. Each ampoule contains: 70% phosphatidylcholine (250 mg), unsaturated fatty acids, vitamin B6, adenosine -5'-monophosphoric acid, nicotinic acid, and benzyl alcohol (preservative). Sanofi-Aventis also offers an oral form called Essentiale. In 1966, Kroupa reported the use of Lipostabil to prevent fat embolism.[57] Lipostabil has been shown to restore the normal equilibrium between low-density lipoprotein (LDL) and high-density lipoprotein (HDL) levels in the blood and to promote cholesterol transport.[49] Based on these findings, in Europe, Lipostabil is indicated for treating hyperlipidemia, atherosclerotic disorders, diabetic angiopathies, angina pectoris, postmyocardial infarction, hypertension of sclerotic origin, and thromboembolism pre- and postoperatively.[58,59]

The aesthetic applications of injectable phosphatidylcholine evolved from the oral and intravenous use of phosphatidylcholine for treating hyperlipidemia and related disorders. In 1988, Maggiori reported the first use of phosphatidylcholine for aesthetic purposes when he used it to treat xanthelasmas.[60] Following Maggiori's report, the use of phosphatidylcholine injections expanded to include subcutaneous injections.

INJECTION LIPOLYSIS USING PHOSPHATIDYLCHOLINE TO REDUCE SUBCUTANEOUS FAT

In 2001, Rittes, a physician practicing in Brazil, first reported in the English dermatologic literature on the subcutaneous injection of phosphatidylcholine to reduce the size of infraorbital fat pads.[61] Thirty patients were studied. The longest follow-up was 2 years. Twenty milligrams of phosphatidylcholine were injected into the central, medial, and lateral fat pads; the distribution per fat pad varied according to the patient's needs. The patients received additional treatments at 15-day intervals if bulging fat pads persisted after the first treatment. Two patients received four treatments; five patients received three treatments. Twelve patients received two treatments, and 11 patients received one treatment. Improvement was noted by observation, and cosmetic improvement was noted in all patients. After treatment, patients noted mild burning that lasted 15 minutes. Edema of the entire lower eyelid lasted approximately 72 hours. There were no reported recurrences.

Other clinical reports soon followed. In 2004, Ablon and Rotunda reported on the use of phosphatidylcholine for treating lower eyelid fat pads; 7 of 10 patients demonstrated a clinical benefit.[62] In 2006, Hasengschwandtner reported on the treatment of 441 patients by injection lipolysis.[63] The patients received a maximum of 2500 mg of phosphatidylcholine per session in a single specific area; the number of sessions varied. One injection contained 0.5 cc of mixture at a depth of 12 mm and 1.5 cm apart; the mixture consisted of phosphatidylcholine 50 mg/mL, NaCl as dilutant, buflomedil (vasodilator) and B-vitamin complex. Pre- and post-treatment circumferences were measured and before and after photographs taken. Post-treatment assessment was made at 8 weeks. Fifteen percent of patients were satisfied after one treatment and 72% after two treatments. The average circumferential reduction was 3.7 cm on the upper belly, 3.9 cm on the lower belly, 1.9 cm on the hips, and 1.6 cm on the upper arm.

SAFETY OF SUBCUTANEOUS INJECTION OF PHOSPHATIDYLCHOLINE

Phosphatidylcholine has been used for many years for preventing and treating fat embolism (intravenous), severe liver failure (oral and intravenous), and in surfactant preparations. Using intravenous and oral phosphatidylcholine preparations for these indications, no significant toxicity is noted even at relatively high doses. The known systemic adverse effects of subcutaneous injection of phosphatidylcholine are cholinergic GI effects including nausea, increased salivation, and abdominal pain. Most practitioners recommend limiting the dose to 2500 mg per treatment session to minimize these effects. These symptoms are similar to the known effects of oral and intravenous phosphatidylcholine-containing preparations. Subcutaneous injections of phosphatidylcholine are associated with burning, urticaria, erythema, swelling, ecchymosis, and pruritis.[64,65] Injections placed too superficially may cause skin ulceration.

One potential outcome after subcutaneous injection with phosphatidylcholine is an efflux of free fatty acids. Free fatty acids are known to cause experimental myocardial infarction in dogs, fat embolism, and steatosis of the liver (A Matarasso and J Kral, personal communication, 2002). Additional concerns center on the potential creation of high levels of lysophosphatidylcholine, the natural degradation product of phosphatidylcholine. Lysophosphatidylcholine is known to cause hepatic cholestasis, liver enzyme elevation, and intravascular hemolysis.[66]

Serious allergic reactions, such as anaphylaxis, have not been reported. Experienced medical practitioners report local adverse effects such as pain, hematoma, edema, and nodules, which are mild and well tolerated; systemic adverse effects are rare (Rittes, 2007). In Hasengschwandtner's 2006 report, no serious adverse effects or complications were noted. In 31 patients who had normal blood work within 6 months before treatment, total bilirubin and gamma glutamyl transferase were checked 5 days and 8 weeks after treatments. All blood values were within normal limits. All patients reported a small-to-medium level of pain, swelling, and erythema. Deep hematomas also were noted. Patients additionally reported soft stools, and four reported menstrual bleeding outside of the normal menstrual cycle. The skin overlying the treated area was noted to be firm and excess skin contracted.

In 2006, Duncan and Chubaty reported on safety data for injection lipolysis using phosphatidylcholine-based formulas.[67] Data were collected from 75 physicians practicing injection lipolysis in 17 countries; 17,376 patients were treated. There were no reports of bacterial or atypical mycobacterial infections, skin ulceration, dermatitis, or chronic skin irritation. Disappointment with the result was noted in 12% of patients. Transient hyperpigmentation (0.015%), allergic reaction (0.0003%), and persistent pain beyond 2 weeks (0.015%) were infrequent.

MECHANISMS OF LIPOLYSIS

Although some reports show a reduction in fat deposits after subcutaneous injection of phosphatidylcholine and deoxycholate, the mechanism by which this would occur is not understood completely. Furthermore, it is not known whether it is the phosphatidylcholine or deoxycholate alone or a combination of both or neither that is producing the clinical effect. Theoretically, several mechanisms could exist alone or in combination.

For the purposes of understanding its possible mechanism of action in fat reduction, it is important to understand the multiple roles of phosphatidylcholine in the human body. The first is its role in the transport and emulsification of dietary fat.[48,68–70] Phosphatidylcholine is found in bile and acts to promote the emulsification of dietary fat. A necessary step in the digestion of dietary fat occurs when fat globules, which are insoluble in water, are broken down into smaller sizes so that water-soluble digestive enzymes can act on the surface of the fat globule. The phosphatidylcholine molecule has a polar (water-soluble) moiety, choline, and a nonpolar (fat-soluble) moiety, the fatty acids. The fat-soluble portion of the phosphatidylcholine dissolves in the surface layer of the fat globule, with the polar portion projecting outward into the aqueous environment.

The polarity of phosphatidylcholine is important for several reasons. First, because the polar head of the phosphatidylcholine is very soluble in the aqueous fluid, the interfacial tension of the fat globule is decreased, and the fat globule can be broken up into minute particles by the normal agitation that occurs during peristalsis of the intestine. In the digestion of fats, this emulsification of fat can increase the total surface area of dietary fat by 1000 times. Thus, intestinal lipases can act upon a much larger surface area than would be available without emulsification. Intestinal lipases break fat down into monoacylglycerol (glycerol with one fatty acid) and fatty acids.

Second, the polarity of phosphatidylcholine contributes to the three different chemical forms of phosphatidylcholine. The first form is the lipid bilayer, with the hydrophobic tail in the middle of the lipid bilayer. The second is a vesicle or liposome, where the lipid bilayer or monolayer forms a circle creating a hydrophilic interior core. The third is a micelle, where the phosphatidylcholine exists in a single layer, with the hydrophilic heads projecting outward, creating a hydrophobic core. Triglycerides and fatty acids are solubilized and transported in the hydrophobic core of the phosphatidylcholine micelle.

The role of phosphatidylcholine in cholesterol metabolism is also important. Phosphatidylcholine is found in HDL, the apolipoprotein that carries fatty acids and cholesterol from the peripheral tissues to the liver. HDLs are so called, because they carry the highest percentage of protein. HDLs exist as spheres with a hydrophic core that is capable of storing cholesterol esters. As more cholesterol is accumulated, the HDL increases in size. Thus, in evaluating risk of atherosclerotic heart disease, it is the ratio of large HDL particles (those that contain more cholesterol) to total HDL that is important.

THE ROLE OF DEOXYCHOLATE (DEOXYCHOLIC ACID)

Phosphatidylcholine alone is very viscous and thus not amenable to injection. For this reason, and as is the case with other injectable pharmaceuticals, sodium deoxycholate, a bile salt, is added to solubilize the phosphatidylcholine, thus making the phosphatidylcholine suitable for injection. Debate exists as to which of the injected chemicals is responsible for the noted clinical results in patients treated for subcutaneous fat reduction. Until recently, it was assumed that the active ingredient in the injectable preparations used for subcutaneous fat reduction was the phosphatidylcholine. Recent data, however, suggest that the sodium deoxycholate also may be an active ingredient that causes cell lysis, which may lead to a reduction in subcutaneous fat, and not just a solubilizing agent.[71] In addition, deoxycholate without phosphatidylcholine has been shown to reduce lipomas.[72] This is further evidence that deoxycholate may play an active role in reducing subcutaneous fat.

Brown discussed the possible role of deoxycholate in injection lipolysis in a 2006 publication.[73] Brown believes that at the concentration used in Lipostabil, deoxycholate would exist as a monomer if injected alone. When injected with phosphatidylcholine into the subcutaneous tissue, four distinct forms of deoxycholate could exist: micelles, vesicles with excess deoxycholate present as monomers, and crystals. It is not known which of these forms is acting on the adipocyte. Brown theorizes that several possibilities could exist:

- Deoxycholate in vesicle form with excess monomers; the monomers lead to cellular necrosis
- Deoxycholate is presented in micelle form, which could result in a mobilization of fat from the adipocyte
- Crystals that are known to be damaging to cells

ADDING IT ALL UP—POSSIBLE MECHANISMS OF ACTION

The current theory is that the clinically observed reduction in subcutaneous fat after injection lipolysis is caused in part by cell wall destruction of the adipocyte followed by a reduction in adipocyte fat. It is possible that either the phosphatidylcholine or deoxycholate or both could be responsible for cell wall destruction. Duncan has shown adipocyte cell wall destruction after injection with compounds containing phosphatidylcholine and deoxycholate.[74] It is thought that the disruption of the adipocyte cell membrane primarily is caused primarily by the deoxycholate contained in the mixture, although phosphatidylcholine alone has been shown to disrupt cell walls.[75]

Following cell wall destruction, there are several possible mechanisms that could lead to reduced volume of fat stored in adipocytes. One possibility is the injected phosphatidylcholine acts to emulsify the stored triglycerides, which then are transported to the liver, where they are metabolized. Duncan showed in one patient injected with phosphatidylcholine containing formula that, after biopsy, the treated area showed cell wall disruption and a reduction in adipocyte diameter. Inflammation and new collagen deposition also were noted. Because fat is stored in adipocytes in the form of triglycerides, it is possible that the smaller adipocyte diameter is caused by transport of triglycerides and fatty acids out of the adipocyte. Theoretically, phosphatidylcholine could dissolve the triglycerides and transport them elsewhere as micelles. The inflammation and new collagen deposition Duncan noted could contribute to the skin tightening noted in treated subjects. Others speculate that after the cell membrane of the adipocyte is disrupted, lipase is activated and breaks down the intracellular fats.

Another possibility is that even if cell wall destruction does not occur, the injected phosphatidylcholine activates lipases, which break down triglycerides to fatty acids, which then are transported as lipoproteins. Phosphatidylcholine also may exert its effect by stimulating beta-receptors or inhibiting alpha-2 receptors, thus producing increased lipolysis activity. Lastly, concentrated amounts of phosphatidylcholine injected subcutaneously could act to emulsify fat, allowing tissue lipases to hydrolyze fat, producing glycerol and free fatty acids.

CONTROVERSIES IN INJECTION LIPOLYSIS

Limited scientific data are available about injection lipolysis. Medical professionals and organizations including the American Society of Plastic Surgeons (ASPS) and the American Society for Aesthetic Plastic Surgery (ASAPS) have criticized the clinical use of phosphatidylcholine and deoxycholate for subcutaneous fat reduction. Among other reasons, there is concern that the clinical application of subcutaneous injection of phosphatidylcholine and deoxycholate preceded IRB-approved studies. Both the ASPS and the ASAPS have issued press releases warning the general public to be wary of mesotherapy until safety and efficacy have been proven.[76,77] The ASAPS issued a position statement that contains recommendations for aesthetic society members regarding mesotherapy and injection lipolysis. In the 2007 position statement, members were advised to "refrain from adopting these treatments until the results of the Aesthetic Surgery Education and Research Foundation (ASERF)-sponsored study are available to provide proof of safety and efficacy, or lack thereof".[78]

Furthermore, the products remain unapproved by the FDA for subcutaneous injection. Lipostabil is not a registered drug in the United States and is not approved by the FDA in the United States for any use. The FDA's current position is that Lipostabil is a new drug under the Federal Food, Drug and Cosmetic Act and thus requires that a new drug application be filed with the FDA before marketing. In addition, no pharmaceutical is approved by the FDA for use in mesotherapy or injection lipolysis for reduction of subcutaneous fat. Practitioners are cautioned to inquire with their malpractice insurance carriers to determine whether mesotherapy or subcutaneous injections using non-FDA approved medications is covered under the terms of their malpractice insurance policy. The use of any of these agents for non-FDA approved indications such as localized fat reduction may place the practitioner at some legal and regulatory risk.[79,80]

The extensive marketing of nonapproved products and treatments is a source of concern in the medical community. Subsequent to the first reports in 2001 on the use of Lipostabil in aesthetic applications, Lipostabil has been marketed around the world under many names including Flabjab and Lipomelt. Other formulas containing phosphatidylcholine and deoxycholate for subcutaneous injection, such as Lipodissolve, also have been marketed aggressively in the United States. The marketing by businesses promoting these products and procedures preceded FDA-approved trials to evaluate the safety and efficacy of these treatments; as such, this marketing was done without documentation of the results claimed or the identification of potential complications. In 2007, the Kansas State Board of Healing Arts, in a ruling that later was overturned, banned all commercial use of Lipodissolve, a compound containing phosphatidylcholine used to reduce subcutaneous fat. The board voted to allow the use of the drug only as part of FDA-sanctioned clinical trials under an investigational new drug application.[81] The company promoting Lipodissolve since has declared bankruptcy. Recently, the name Lipodissolve was trademarked by a nonphysician who offers courses on the lipodissolve technique. Furthermore, in the United States, it is illegal to advertise the use of an unapproved product or an off-label use of an approved product. Although the enforcement of these regulations may seem lax, practitioners are exposed to enforcement actions by the FDA, actions by state medical boards, and other sanctions.

To date, there are no published IRB-approved trials evaluating the subcutaneous injection of phosphatidylcholine and deoxycholate. One such study recently began and, as of this writing, has several patients enrolled. In early July 2008, Dr. V. Leroy Young, after obtaining an investigational new drug (IND) permit from the FDA, began an IRB-approved study evaluating the effects of the subcutaneous injection of phosphatidylcholine and deoxycholate (TM Pfeifer and Young VL, personal communication, 2008). The study is sponsored by the Aesthetic Surgery Education and Research Foundation of ASAPS. It is overseen by the Western IRB and the IRB of Washington University. Early study results are anticipated in March 2009.

SUMMARY

Localized deposits of excess adipose tissue and indeed obesity can be medically dangerous and psychologically distressing to patients. With respect to mesotherapy as a method of body contouring, more studies are necessary before advocating this as a safe and effective treatment. Physicians practicing injection lipolysis are working to elucidate the safety and efficacy of the subcutaneous injection of phosphatidylcholine and deoxycholate.[82] Finally, establishing standards of practice to ensure patient safety is an absolute priority for these physicians.

The lipolysis responsible for reduced subcutaneous fat after injection lipolysis may result in increased levels of free fatty acids and glycerol in the bloodstream. To ensure the safety of injection lipolysis with phosphatidylcholine and deoxycholate, it would be prudent to know the products of dissolution, whether free fatty acids are released into the patient's bloodstream, whether the injected chemical is absorbed into the bloodstream, the effects on the liver and other organs, the appropriate dose, among other things. Moreover, although the intracellular contents of the adipocyte can be reduced, the fate of the adipose cell membrane and how that may affect recurrence are unknown.

When skillfully applied to the appropriate patient, the results of body-contouring procedures are pleasing to the plastic surgeon and patient. The promise of a simple, permanent method of reducing subcutaneous fat is obviously very appealing. In view of cultural attitudes that value a trim physique and youthful appearance and the rise in the number of overweight individuals in society, it is likely that the demand for body-contouring procedures including liposuction and other potential methods such as mesotherapy and injection lipolysis will increase. Physicians must strive to evaluate new treatment modalities through rigorous scientific study while at the same time keeping an open mind about potential new therapies that could benefit patients.

REFERENCES

1. Pistor M. [What is mesotherapy?] [abstract]. Chir Dent Fr 1976;46:59.
2. Petit P. The history of mesotherapy. In: Madhere, editor. Aesthetic mesotherapy and injection lipolysis in clinical practice. Informa Healthcare; 2007. p. 20.
3. Available at: www.caringmedical.com/therapies/mesotherapy.asp. October 2003.
4. Weekend Mag 2001.
5. People Magazine 2003.
6. Le Coz J. Traité de Mésotherapie. Masson; 2005.
7. Le Coz J. Mesotherapy and lipolysis: a comprehensive clinical approach. France: Esthetic Medic; 2008.
8. Aesthetic mesotherapy and injection lipolysis in clinical practice. Madhère, editor.
9. Available at: http://www.usameso.com. Accessed June 23, 2008.
10. Medioni G. Results of 6 years of treatment of painful periodontal episodes by mesotherapy. Chir Dent Fr 1980;46:97.
11. Dalloz-Bourguignon A. A new therapy against pain: mesotherapy. J Belge Med Phys Rehabil 1979;2:230.
12. Vaillant P. Remission of painful oro-dental symptoms using treatment with mesotherapy. Chir Dent Fr 1986;56:41.
13. Donini I, DeAnna D, Carella G, et al. Mesotherapy in the treatment of lymphedema: histologic and ultrastructural observations. Chir Patol Sper 1982;30:25.
14. Gallo R. Mesotherapy in phlebology. Phlebologie 1980;33:153.
15. Menkes CJ, Laoussadi S, Kac-Ohana N, et al. Controlled trial of injectable diclofenac in mesotherapy for the treatment of tendonitis. Rev Rhum Mal Osteoartic 1990;57:589.
16. Soncini G, Costantino C. The treatment of pathologic calcification of shoulder tendons with E.D.T.A. bisodum salt by mesotherapy. Acta Biomed Ateneo Parmense 1998;69:133.
17. Guazzetti R, Iotti E, Marinoni E. Mesotherapy with naproxin sodium in musculoskeletal disease. Riv Eur Sci Med Farmacol 1988;10:539.
18. Brule-Fermand S. Treatment of chronic cancer pain. Contribution of acupuncture, auriculotherapy, and mesotherapy. Soins 1993;568:39.
19. Kalil A. Aesthetic mesotherapy: the US approach and contribution. J Cosmet Dermatol 2006;19:753.
20. Davis MD, Wright TI, Shehan JM. A complication of mesotherapy: noninfectious granulomatous panniculitis. Arch Dermatol 2008;144:808.
21. Al-Khenaizan S. Facial cutaneous ulcers following mesotherapy. Dermatol Surg 2008;34:832.
22. Kadry R, Hamadah I, Al-Issa A, et al. Multifocal scalp abscess with subcutaneous fat necrosis and scarring alopecia as a complication of scalp mesotherapy. J Drugs Dermatol 2008;7:72.
23. Munayco CV, Grijalva CG, Culqui DR, et al. Outbreak of persistant cutaneous abscesses due to Mycobacterium chelonae after mesotherapy sessions. Lima (Peru), Peru. Rev Saude Publica 2008;42:146
24. Sañudo A, Vallejo F, Sierra M, et al. Nontuberculous mycobacteria infection after mesotherapy: preliminary report of 15 cases. Int J Dermatol 2007;46:649.
25. Brandão C, Fernandes N, Mesquita N, et al. Abdominal hematoma—a mesotherapy complication. Acta Derm Venereol 2005;85:446.
26. Bessis D, Guilhou JJ, Guillot B. Localized urticaria pigmentosa triggered by mesotherapy. Dermatology 2004;209:343.
27. Rosina P, Chieregato C, Miccolis D, et al. Psoriasis and side effects of mesotherapy. Int J Dermatol 2001;40:581.
28. Nagore E, Ramos P, Botells-Estrada R, et al. Cutaneous infection with Mycobacterium fortuitum after localized microinjections (mesotherapy) treated successfully with a triple drug regimen. Acta Derm Venereol 2001;81:291–3.
29. Urbani CE. Urticarial reaction to ethylenediamine in aminophylline following mesotherapy. Contact Derm 1994;31:198.
30. Paul C, Burguiere AM, Vincent V, et al. [BCG-induced mycobacterium infection induced by alternative medicine.]. Ann Dermatol Venereol 1997;124:710.
31. Marco-Bonnet J, Beylot-Barry M, Texier-Maugein J, et al. [Mycobacterial bovis BCG cutaneous

infections following mesotherapy: 2 cases]. Ann Dermatol Venereol 2007;129:728.

32. Ordiz I. Tratado de Mesoterapia. Oviedo: KRK; 2000.

33. Available at: http://mesoestheticusa.com/contacto.html. Accessed July 2, 2008.

34. Matarasso A. Ultrasonic assisted liposucton: is this new technology for you. Clin Plast Surg 1999; 26(3):369.

35. Medicamento Lipostabil não possui registro no Brasil. Available at: http://www.lipotreatmentfacts.org/downloads/AnvisaNotmcias.pdf. Accessed June 23, 2008.

36. Pharmacy creations, compounding, and nutritional pharmacy. Randolf, NJ.

37. Rutunda AM, Kolodney MS. Mesotherapy and phosphatidylcholine injections: historical clarification and review. Dermatol Surg 2006;32:465.

38. Park SH, Kim DW, Lee MA, et al. Effectiveness of mesotherapy on body contouring. Plast Reconstr Surg 2008;121:179e.

39. Greenway FL, Bray GA, Heber D. Topical fat reduction. Obes Res 1995;3(Suppl 4):561S.

40. Greenway FL, Bray GA. Regional fat loss from the thigh in obese women after adrenergic modulation. Clin Ther 1987;9:663.

41. Salas AP, Asaadi M. Aesthetic application of mesotherapy: a preliminary report [Abstract Presented at the Annual Meeting of the American Society of Aesthetic Plastic Surgery]. Vancouver, British Columbia, April 17, 2004.

42. Velasco MF, Tano CT, Machado-Santelli GM, et al. Effects of caffeine and siloxanetriol alginate caffeine, as anticellulite agents, on fatty tissue: histological evaluation. J Cosmet Dermatol 2008;7:23.

43. Morimoto C, Kameda K, Tsujita T, et al. Relationships between lipolysis induced by various lipolytic agents and hormone-sensitive lipase in rat fat cells. J Lipid Res 2001;42:120.

44. Borsheim E, Lonnroth P, Knarkahl S, et al. No difference in the lipolytic response to beta-adrenoreceptor stimulation in situ but a delayed increase in adipose tissue blood flow in moderately obese compared with lean men the postexercise period. Metamedicine 2000;49:579.

45. Kolehmainen M, Ohisalo JJ, Kaartenen JM, et al. Concordance of in vivo microdialysis and in vitro techniques in the studies of adipose tissue metabolism. Int J Obes Relat Metab Disord 2000;24:1426.

46. Caruso MK, Roberts AT, Bissoon L, et al. An evaluation of mesotherapy solutions for inducing lipolysis and treating cellulite. J Plast Reconstr Aesthet Surg 2007.

47. Rosenbaum M, Prieto V, Hellmer J, et al. An exploratory investigation of the morphology and biochemistry of cellulite. Plast Reconstr Surg 1998;101:1934.

48. Lehninger AC, Neslon DL, Cox MM. Lipid biosynthesis. In: Principles of biochemistry. 9th edition. New York: Worth Publishers; 1993. p. 642.

49. Almazov VA, Freidlin IS, Krasil'nikova EI. The use of lipostabil to correct lipid metabolism disorder in patients with ischemic heart disease. Kardiologiia 1986;26:39.

50. Levy R. Lecithin in Alzheimer's disease. Lancet 1982;2:671.

51. Young VL. Lipostabil: the effect of phosphatidylcholine on subcutaneous fat. Aesthet Surg J 2003;23:413.

52. Polichetti E, Jannisson A, de la Porte PL, et al. Dietary polyenylphosphatidylcholine decreases cholesterolemia in hypercholesterolemic rabbits: role of the hepato-biliary axis. Life Sci 2000;67:2563.

53. Navder KP, Lieber CS. Dilinoleoylphosphatidylcholine is responsible for the beneficial effects of plyenylphosphatidylcholine on ethanol-induced mitochondrial injury in rats. Biochem Biophys Res Commun 2002;8:1109.

54. Mi LJ, Mak KM, Lieber CS. Attenuation of alcohol-induced apoptosis of hepatocytes in rat livers by polyenylphosphatidylcholine (PPC). Alcohol Clin Exp Res 2000;24:207.

55. Navder KP, Baraona E, Lieber CS. Polyenylphosphatidylcholine decreases alcoholic hyperlipemia without affecting the alcohol-induced rise of HDL-cholesterol. Life Sci 1997;61:1907.

56. Aleynik SI, Leo MA, Ma X, et al. Plyenylphosphatidylcholine prevents carbon tetrachloride-induced lipid peroxidation while it attenuates liver fibrosis. J Hepatol 1997;27:554.

57. Kroupa J. The role of pharmacology in the comprehensive prophylaxis of post-traumatic fat embolism. Acta Chir Orthop Traumatol Cech 1993;60:114.

58. Lipostabil package insert. Aventis Pharma, January 11, 2001.

59. Mel'chinskaia EN, Fromnatskii NI, Kirichenko LL. Hypolipidemic effects of alisat and lipostabil in patients with diabetes mellitus. Ter Arkh 2000;72:57.

60. Maggiori S. Treatment of xanthelasma with phosphatidylcholine. Presented at the 5th International Meeting of Mesotherapy. Paris, France, 1988.

61. Rittes PG. The use of phosphatidylcholine for correction of lower lid bulging due to prominent fat pads. Dermatol Surg 2001;27:391.

62. Ablon G, Rotunda AM. Treatment of lower eyelid fat pads using phosphatidylcholine: clinical trial and review. Dermatol Surg 2004;30:422.

63. Hasengschwandtner F. Injection lipolysis for effective reductin of localized fat in place of minor surgical lipoplasty. Aesthet Surg J 2006;26:125.

64. Hexsel D, Serra M, Mazzuco R, et al. Phosphatidylcholine in the treatment of localized fat. J Drugs Dermatol 2003;2:511.

65. Palmer M, Curran J, Bowler P. Clinical experience and safety using phosphatidylcholine injections for

the localized reduction of subcutaneous fat: a multe-centre, retrospective UK study. J Cosmet Dermatol 2006;5:218.

66. Teelmann K, Schlappi B, Schupbach M, et al. Preclinical safety evaluation of intravenously administered mixed micelles. Arzneimittelforschung 1984; 34:1517.

67. Duncan DI, Chubaty R. Clinical safety data and standards of practice for injection lipolysis: a retrospective study. Aesthet Surg J 2006;26:575.

68. Tso P, Crissinger K. Digestion and absorption of lipids. In: Stipanuck MH, editor. Biochemical and physiological aspects of human nutrition. Philadelphia: W.B. Saunders; 2000. p. 125.

69. Guyton AC, Hall JE. Lipid metabolism. In: Textbook of medical physiology. 9th edition. Philadelphia: W.B. Saunders; 1996. p. 865.

70. Bhagavan NV. Lipids II: phospholipids, glycocphingolipids, and cholesterol. In: Medical biochemistry. 4th edition. San Diego (CA): Harcourt Academic Press; 2002. p. 401.

71. Rotunda AM, Suzuki H, Moy RL, et al. Detergent effects of sodium deoxycholate are a major feature of an injectable phosphatidylcholine formulation used for localized fat dissolution. Dermatol Surg 2004;30:1001.

72. Rotunda AM, Ablon G, Kilodney MS. Lipomas treated with subcutaneous injections of sodium deoxycholate. J Am Acad Dermatol 2005;53:973.

73. Brown SA. The science of mesotherapy: chemical anarchy. Aesthet Surg J 2006;26:95.

74. Duncan DI. Lipodissolve for subcutaneous fat reduction and skin retraction. Aesthet Surg J 2005; 25:530.

75. Hasengschwandtner F. Phosphatidylcholine treatment to induce lipolysis. J Cosmet Dermatol 2005; 4:308.

76. Mesotherapy not proven as a safe alternative to liposuction. Available at: http://www.plasticsurgery. org/media/press_releases/Mesotherapy-Not-Proven-As-A-Safe-Alternative-to-Liposuction.cfm. Accessed June 20, 2008.

77. Fat-melting fad: too good to be true?. ASAPS news release; 2004.

78. The American Society for Aesthetic Plastic Surgery's position statement on injection lipolysis (lipodissolve or mesotherapy). Available at: http://www. surgery.org/members/whatsnew-052007.php. Accessed June 20, 2008.

79. Aicher R. Cosmetic surgery and the law. The American Society for Aesthetic Plastic Surgery. The Aesthetic Society News 2003;7:11.

80. Rohrich RJ, Jeffrey EJ, Reisman NR. Use of off-label and nonapproved drugs and devices in plastic surgery. Plast Reconstr Surg 2003;112:241.

81. Available at: http://www.bizjournals.com/stlouis/ stories/2007/09/10/daily64.html. Accessed February 3, 2008.

82. Duncan DI, Palmer P. Fat reduction using phosphatidylcholine/sodium deoxycholate injections: standard of practice. Aesthetic Plast Surg, accepted for publication.

Comment on "Mesotherapy and Injection Lipolysis"

Jack A. Friedland, MD

KEYWORDS
- Mesotherapy • Injection lipolysis
- Subcutaneous fat reduction
- Non-surgical body contour improvement

The authors of "Mesotherapy and Injection Lipolysis" state that the purpose of their article is to familiarize readers with the evolution of mesotherapy, injection lipolysis, and the use of phosphatidylcholine and deoxycholate for subcutaneous fat reduction. The clinical application of mesotherapy was not preceded by rigorous scientific study of the chemicals and their use, which is necessary to establish their safety and efficacy. The process and the formulas have not been approved by the US Food and Drug Administration.

The evolution of mesotherapy for reducing subcutaneous fat and improving body contour is reviewed by the authors in great detail. Opinion differs regarding the various formulas and ingredients, and a debate exists within the community of mesotherapy practitioners as to which techniques are most appropriate. Differences exist regarding exactly where, how much, and how often the chemicals are to be injected. This lack of standardized formulas and protocols makes it virtually impossible to validate results and compare reports of efficacy. In addition, many complications and side effects from the treatments have been reported. Although some practitioners of mesotherapy are properly trained in medicine, in many countries, including the United States, unlicensed or unsupervised practitioners are providing treatments. These individuals may not be properly trained, and more often than not they do not have the ability to fully evaluate a patient's condition or offer appropriate alternative treatments necessary to care for complications. In addition, mesotherapy injections contain ingredients that are inexpensive and easily obtainable, and the solutions used may not be standardized or even completely sterile.

The promise of a simple nonsurgical, noninvasive, permanent method of reducing subcutaneous fat is very appealing. I do not believe that mesotherapy should be considered as an alternative to surgical liposuction. When mesotherapy is used in conjunction with dietary modification, hormone replacement, exercise, and nutritional supplements, the attribution of the results from mesotherapy (any reduction of subcutaneous fat) is difficult to precisely identify. "Mesotherapy and Injection Lipolysis" thoroughly reviews the research that has been done to clarify mechanisms by which mesotherapy might possibly work, but the reduction of fat deposits after subcutaneous injections is not completely understood.

As physicians, we must strive to evaluate new treatment modalities through rigorous scientific study, while at the same time keeping an open mind about potential new therapies that could benefit patients. This article by Drs. Matarasso and Pfeifer is one of the most extensive, yet most easily understandable reviews of this subject, and it should be required reading for all plastic surgeons who perform procedures for body contour improvement.

7425 East Shea Boulevard, Suite 103, Scottsdale, AZ 85260–6411, USA
E-mail address: jaf@jackafriedlandmd.com

Clin Plastic Surg 36 (2009) 193
doi:10.1016/j.cps.2008.11.012

Refinement of Technique in Injection Lipolysis Based on Scientific Studies and Clinical Evaluation

Diane Duncan, MD, FACS[a],*, J. Peter Rubin, MD[b], Loren Golitz, MD[c], Stephen Badylak, DVM, MD, PhD[b], Lynne Kesel, DVM[d], John Freund, BS[b], Danielle Duncan[e]

KEYWORDS

- Injection lipolysis • Mesotherapy • Phosphatidylcholine
- Sodium deoxycholate • Stem cell study • Skin retraction

Although the practice of mesotherapy dates to 2000 BC,[1] the specific use of injections targeted to reduce subcutaneous fat is relatively new. Injection lipolysis is not considered mesotherapy.[2] Mesotherapy is an alternative medicine practice in which microinjections of various pharmaceuticals are injected in particular regions of the body in order to treat specific conditions that can range from sports injuries to systemic illnesses, alopecia, gynecologic dysfunction, and even nicotine dependence. The drugs are mixed as a cocktail, and in many instances, the recipe varies from one practitioner to another. The injections can be placed in the dermis, subcutaneous fat, or regionally in the intramuscular or carotid sinus area.

In contrast, injection lipolysis has a single target: subcutaneous fat. Although the injectable substance varies slightly, the formula usually contains a combination of phosphatidylcholine and sodium deoxycholate.[3] The practice of fat reduction with PC/DC has been studied clinically for 13 years,[4] but few scientific studies have been performed in a laboratory setting. Animal studies are rare.[5] Although several histopathology slides are featured in clinical articles, no serial changes over time have been published. Once the mechanism of action is understood, the potential use and limitations of the treatment can be delineated better.

DEFINING LIPOLYSIS

Although many patients and physicians believe that lipolysis always means permanent destruction of fat cells, there are two situations in which the use of of the term "lipolysis" is appropriate. The physiologic basis of the commonly used term lipolysis can be a result of either the fight-or-flight mechanism,[6] or it can mean permanent cell wall lysis leading to necrosis. Although the egress of glycerol and free fatty acids from adipocytes into the bloodstream is stimulated by epinephrine, norepinephrine, and isoproterenol, the fat cells themselves are not necessarily damaged by that process. In fact, when the crisis is over, most of the fatty elements that were mobilized to provide energy move back into the adipocytes. In order to induce enough damage to the cell to cause necrosis, a large enough section of the cell membrane must be damaged so that the cell cannot repair itself. A more accurate term to define

[a] Private Practice, Ft. Collins, CO, USA
[b] University of Pittsburgh, Pittsburgh, PA, USA
[c] Univeristy of Colorado, Denver, CO, USA
[d] Colorado State University, Fort Collins, CO, USA
[e] University of Colorado, Boulder, CO, USA
* Corresponding author.
E-mail address: momsurg@aol.com (D. Duncan).

Clin Plastic Surg 36 (2009) 195–209
doi:10.1016/j.cps.2008.11.001
0094-1298/08/$ – see front matter © 2009 Published by Elsevier Inc.

the goal of nonsurgical fat reduction might be adipocyte lysis or fat necrosis. Neither of these terms is as marketable as lipodissolve or even injection lipolysis. Yet the goal in reducing a localized fat deposit is a permanent reduction in size, degree of protrusion, degree of skin laxity, irregularity in contour, and reduction of unsightly bulges and overhang when the patient is wearing certain types of clothing.

Many mesotherapists use beta-adrenergic drugs as part of their cocktails, hoping to stimulate fat loss with green tea extract, aminophylline, or caffeine injected into the fat. Although almost all patients experience some adverse effects from these substances, there is as yet no scientific data that support permanent fat reduction caused by the use of beta-adrenergic drugs in an injectable fat-reducing formula.

ACHIEVING PERMANENT FAT REDUCTION

The Federal Trade Commission commissioned a study in 2004[7] showing that 95% to 98% of commercial diets fail. Americans spend over $55 billion yearly trying to lose weight and fat. This study, geared toward truth in advertising, also found that although exercising is an excellent way to maintain muscle tone and reduce stress, the use of exercise alone as a weight loss tool was ineffective.

Most physicians know that sit-ups will not create a flat abdomen, and the "Lovehandler"[8] will not get rid of localized fat in the flank region.

The only solution for permanent fat reduction in these genetically and hormonally driven localized fat deposits is either the physical removal or induction of necrosis of the adipocytes in the targeted region. Six methods for inducing physical disruption of cells exist in the research laboratory.[9] These include: mechanical grinding, liquid homogenization, sonication, use of a freeze/thaw cycle, manual grinding or avulsion, and the use of detergents to chemically induce cell wall disruption. The Waring blender is the time-honored way to reduce a large piece of tissue into a more workable form. The French press, which uses a piston to push a volume of tissue through a small hole in the press, works well at homogenizing tissue. Although neither of these methods can be applied to living organisms, the original method of liposuction closely approximates these physically destructive modalities. Sonication—the application of pulsed high frequency ultrasound waves to tissue in solution—shears the cell walls. The use of a freeze/thaw cycle works when ice crystals form within the cell, causing swelling and subsequent disruption from the inside of the cell. Manual

grinding can be done with glass beads or mortar and pestle in the laboratory, but this method has no real application in people. Manual avulsion is a more effective method and is used in suction assisted lipectomy.

The use of detergents is a milder solution to achieving cell lysis in many cases. The mechanism of action is that detergents "break the lipid barrier surrounding cells by solubilizing proteins and disrupting lipid:lipid, protein:protein, and protein:lipid interactions."[10] The behavior of the detergent depends on the molecular properties of the head and the tail of the detergent molecule; detergents can be inonic (cationic or anionic), zwitterionic, or nonionic.[11] Usually the milder detergents are nonionic or zwitterionic. Fewer proteins are denatured when these mild detergents are used. Ionic detergents—both anionic and cationic—tend to be a little harsher. Sodium deoxycholate, the detergent used as a solvent to dissolve the solid phosphatidylcholine into solution, is a milder ionic detergent than many other commercial detergents. Animal cells are complex and frequently require both chemical and physical elements in order to induce permanent cell wall lysis. Other elements that may help improve the degree of cell lysis are the use of a buffer, manipulation of tissue temperature, solution viscosity and dispersion characteristics, pH, and salinity of the solution.

SERIAL HISTOLOGY STUDY

Many suppositions and proposed mechanisms of action for injection lipolysis have been presented at meetings and published in the medical literature over the past 4 years.[12–14] Publications have included isolated histology slides, but none have examined the progression of the changes in the subcutaneous tissue at and near the injection sites.[15,16]

Six patient volunteers desiring extra fat reduction and skin retraction in the abdominal region were treated with phosphatidylcholine 50 mg/mL and sodium deoxycholate 42 mg/mL at 1 hour, 1 day, 1 week, 2 weeks, 3 weeks, and 4 weeks before their scheduled abdominoplasty. These patients all had a centrally located lipodystrophy extending into the supraumbilical region.

Those included for the study were: female patients between the ages of 25 and 60, with a postpartum deformity including periumbilical lipodystrophy, diastasis recti, mild-to-moderate skin laxity, a body mass index (BMI) of 28 or less, and a desire for dramatic contour correction.

Patients excluded were women who were or might possibly be pregnant, women who were lactating, patients with an allergy or sensitivity to soy products, those who had a serious ongoing systemic illness, and women who had an open sore or lesion in the treatment region. No patient was taking ibuprofen, aspirin, or other anticoagulant type medication. None had any conditions that might create a suppression of the immune response.

MATERIALS AND METHODS

Phosphatidylcholine 50 mg/mL with deoxycholate 42 mg/mL, normal saline for injection 0.9%, and plain deoxycholate, 42 mg/mL were obtained from MasterPharm (Richmond Hills, New York). Manual injection following a grid pattern spacing injections 1.5 cm apart was planned. 10 cc syringes were used to draw up and to inject the PC/DC solution. A 26 gauge 3/8 in needle (Becton and Dickinson, Franklin Lakes, New Jersey) was used to inject the solution to a uniform superficial depth. To evaluate the activity of unbuffered detergent, a single injection of 0.4 cc deoxycholate 42 mg/mL without the phosphatidylcholine was planned in the region just below the umbilicus, which would be removed at the time of abdominoplasty. Pc 50/ DC 42 and normal saline as a control were tested in a similar manner.

Standard preoperative photographs were performed, and an informed study consent was obtained. The patients were all treated with injection lipolysis before their surgical abdominoplasty procedure.

The procedure for the injections included a history and physical examination. Close attention was given to examination of the treatment region. Each patient was asked to circle, with a sterile marking pen, the region of the abdomen she disliked most. All six of the women drew a guitar-shaped diagram on the abdomen, extending up to the base of the rib cage. Because the infraumbilical region was planned to be resected, injections were given in the supra-and periumbilical region in order to achieve a clinical effect, and in the immediate infraumbilical region in order to produce a small region for biopsy purposes. With the patient's permission, the infraumbilical region that would be resected was tattooed at three points before the three injections in order to positively identify those sites as the injection sites.

The region for epigastric injection was demarcated using a 1.5 cm grid. Sterile preparation of the entire treatment region was performed with chlorhexidine. Using a pinch-and-pull technique, each patient was injected with the phosphatidylcholine50 mg/mL and deoxycholate 42 mg/mL (PC/DC) solution in a 0.4 cc dose per injection site. A total of 26 cc of solution was used for each treatment. The injection site for biopsy was treated with a 0.4 cc injection of PC/DC on the right infraumbilical abdomen, and with deoxycholate alone on the left infraumbilical abdomen. An infraumbilical injection site also was injected with the saline control. The entire region again was cleansed with chlorhexidine following the injections, and a cool compress was applied to the treatment region for 10 minutes.

The interval between the injection sessions and the abdominoplasty varied. One patient was treated 1 hour before surgery, and another received injections 1 day before treatment. The four remaining patients underwent injections at 1 week, 2 weeks, 3 weeks, and 4 weeks before their abdominoplasties.

A 1 cm^2 biopsy of skin and subcutaneous fat was taken at each tattooed site during each patient's abdominoplasty. One biopsy contained tissue treated with PC50/ DC42; one was injected with the saline control, and the other specimen had tissue treated with deoxycholate alone (**Fig. 1**). Specimens were sent to Dr. Loren Golitz, a dermatopathologist practicing in Denver, Colorado, for evaluation.

REACTION OF THE SKIN OVERLYING THE TREATMENT REGION

Despite the fact that only the subcutaneous fat is injected, there is a clear reaction of the skin in the treatment region (**Fig. 2**).

In most cases, some improvement in skin quality can be seen, with mild skin retraction and up to 12% thickening of the dermis, measured with serial micrometry. Occasionally, however, there are instances of prolonged skin discoloration or even skin loss in the treatment region. Histologic evaluation of the dermis in the treatment region was performed in order to better understand what effects injection lipolysis has on the overlying skin. Biopsies were taken as for the subcutaneous fat: at 1 hour, 1 day, 1 week, 2 weeks, 3 weeks, and 4 weeks after injection of a saline control, PC50/DC42, and deoxycholate 4.2%.

SUMMARY OF FINDINGS

The regions injected with a saline control showed no histologic changes other than mild inflammation at any time.

At 1 hour after injection, the phosphatidylcholine/deoxcholate solution produced no visible cytotoxic reaction, while the plain deoxycholate induced massive immediate fat necrosis. A similar pattern was seen with both formulas at 1 day after injection. Fat necrosis appeared at 1 week in small regions with the PC/DC formula.

The deoxycholate specimen began to show immediate and intense inflammatory changes and fibrosis.

At 2 weeks, all four elements of fat necrosis were present in PC/DC specimens: inflammation, neovascularization, fat cell lysis, and macrophage infiltration, as well as thickening of fibrous septae. The deoxycholate specimen showed large regions of "moth-eaten" fat, where no cells were present. At 1 month, the PC/DC specimens still showed

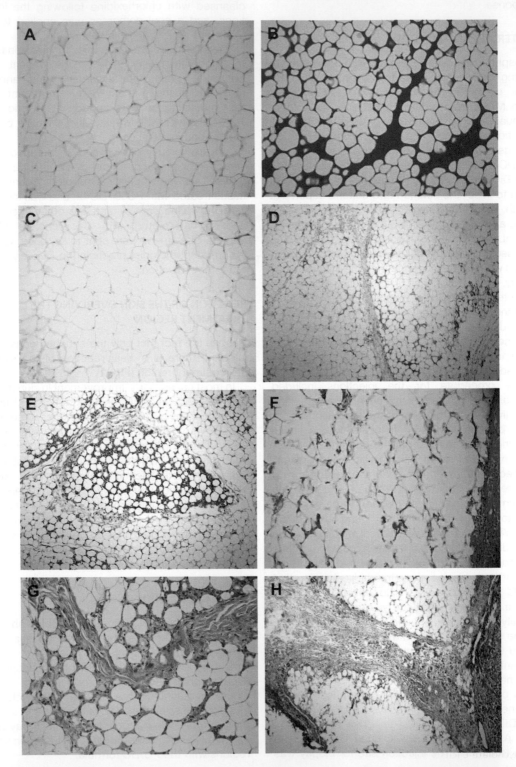

a fractionated response, while the deoxycholate specimens showed a dramatic and extensive eradication of adipose cells with severe fibrotic scarring in the subcutaneous layer.

To date, no description of what happens in the skin overlying the treatment regions has been published. It appears that the PC/DC formula causes a gradual onset of inflammation within the dermis adjacent to the treatment region. The infiltrate is characterized as a sterile cellulitis, as polymorphnuclear leucocytes greatly outnumber lymphocytes. These cells are noted near the deep dermal plexus, and to a lesser extent, near the superficial blood supply of the dermis. The adnexal elements such as eccrine sweat glands, hair follicles, and nerves show inflammation in the PC/DC biopsies late in the course of the healing process. The specimens near the deoxycholate injections showed more intense inflammation at an earlier point than did the PC/DC specimens. Some patchy necrosis of sweat glands, blood vessel walls, and nerves was seen in the deoxycholate specimens at 3 to 4 weeks after injection. Necrobiosis, or degeneration of the basal dermis, was seen in the deoxycholate specimen at 1 month.

STEM CELL STUDY: EFFICACY OF INJECTION LIPOLYSIS COMPONENTS FOR ADIPOCYTE CELL LYSIS
In Vitro

The lipolytic value of each constituent component of the standard PC50/ DC42 formula has been debated for several years.[17,18] The difficulty in testing phosphatidylcholine is that it is impossible to get it into solution without a solvent.

Almost all solvents have a detergent-like effect, solubilizing the lipid bilayer of cell walls. A major challenge of this study was finding a biologically inert solvent so that phosphatidylcholine could be tested by itself. Because this in vitro study required no human injection of the solvent, biologically inactive mineral oil was used, as it was found to dissolve phosphatidylcholine in a 5% solution,

or 50 mg/mL, the standard concentration in the most commonly used lipolysis formulas. The concentration of all other ingredients was calculated at the same strength as used in many commercially available formulas.

The development process for the best lipolytic agent has been difficult. Until recently, Aventis, the makers of Lipostabil, have shown no interest in obtaining Agencia Nacional de Vigilancia Sanitaria (ANVISA) or US Food and Drug Administration (FDA) approval for its use for subcutaneous fat reduction.[19] Kythera (Los Angeles, California) is involved in clinical trials of ATX-101, a lipolytic injectable with a deoxycholate dominant formula.[20] Neither of these drugs has been approved by a licensing body in the United States or abroad for injection for fat reduction. Because injectors can obtain a similar low-cost formulation legally from compounding pharmacies, it may not be cost-effective for a large pharmaceutical firm to go through the expensive and time-consuming FDA approval process for obtaining PC/DC approval.

The purpose on this in vitro study was to evaluate the effect of various constituent components of the injection lipolysis solution on cultured human adipocytes.

Materials and Methods

The study was performed at the McGowan Research Institute in Pittsburgh using human adult-derived adipocytes cultured from stem cells under an approved protocol. Adipose tissue from five human subjects was collected. The cells were fractionated using a collagenase digestion method, yielding preadipocytes, which structurally resemble fibroblasts. The preadipocytes were cultured until near confluence for 2 weeks. They then were differentiated into adipocytes using insulin, dexamethasone, and other growth factors for 14 days. This step provided a healthy and robust cell population on which to test the lipolysis

Fig.1. (A) Subcutaneous fat injected with saline control, 1 day after injection. All saline control photomicrographs appear similar throughout the duration of the study. (B) Subcutaneous fat injected with deoxycholate 4.2%, 1 day after injection. 100% fat necrosis is present. Cells without viable nuclei are surrounded by hyaline ground substance. (C) Fat injected with PC50/ DC42 1 day after injection. Appears very similar to saline control at this point. (D) Subcutaneous fat injected with PC50/ DC42 at 1 week. Note thickening of fibrous septae and fractionated pattern of fat necrosis. (E) Fat injected with PC50/ DC 42 at 2 weeks after injection. Some fat globules have more of a response than others. Fat necrosis, inflammation, and fibrous septae thickening are more prominent. (F) Specimen injected with deoxycholate at 3 weeks after injection. Fat/dermal junction is at right. Note massive cell lysis and inflammation. (G) At 3 weeks after injection with PC 50/ DC42, inflammation, thickening of fibrous septae, and the presence of macrophages are seen. Some viable fat cells are still present. (H) 4 weeks after injection with deoxycholate 4.2%, massive fat necrosis and formation of fibrous tissue are apparent. Unbuffered deoxycholate elicits a dramatic and intense reaction.

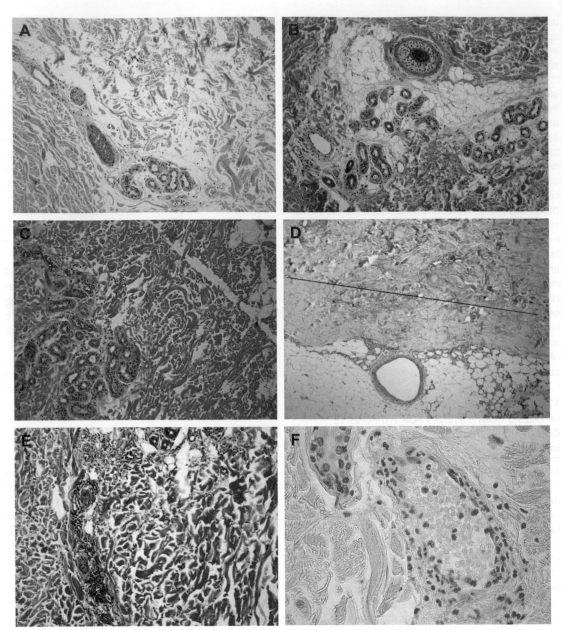

Fig. 2. (*A*) Dermal elements overlying subcutaneous fat injected with saline control at 1 day after injection. Dermal adnexae are normal. A mild, diffuse inflammatory infiltrate is seen. The appearance of the saline control specimens remained similar during the 4 weeks after injection. (*B*) Dermal elements overlying the region treated with deoxycholate 4.2% 1 day after injection. Note profound fat necrosis in the fatty peninsula near the hair follicle. More intense inflammation is present than in the saline specimen, especially near the adnexae. (*C*) Dermal elements, 1 day after injection with PC50/ DC42. Mild inflammation was noted. (*D*) Dermal/fat junction, 3 weeks after deoxycholate injection. The basal layer of the dermis has undergone necrobiosis (below line), a condition in which degenerating collagen acquires a bluish appearance, while the healthy collagen fibers remain bright pink. Patchy necrosis of eccrine glands, nerve sheaths, and blood vessel walls can be seen. This pattern was not noted in the PC/DC specimens. (*E*) Dermis 3 weeks after PC50/ DC42 injection. Inflammation is prominent, but collagen fibers remain bright pink. (*F*) Vasculitis in dermis overlying a region treated with deoxycholate only. This reaction does not occur immediately; it usually appears at 3 to 5 weeks after injection.

components. A fibroblast cell line and vehicle controls were included for all treatments.

For all experiments, the authors obtained adipose tissue from the abdominal subcutaneous region or the thigh subcutaneous region, as these are areas commonly treated with injection lipolysis. Specimens were minced, then digested in a balanced salt solution containing 1 mg/mL collagenase and 3.5% fatty acidfree BSA in a 37° shaking water bath until fragments were no longer visible and the digest had a milky appearance. Digests were filtered, then centrifuged at 1000 rpm for 10 minutes. Floating adipocytes were removed. The remaining cells were treated with an erythrocyte lysis buffer. The resulting preadipocytes were plated using a low-serum plating medium for 6 hours; all unattached cells were discarded.

Preadipocytes were grown to near confluence in plating medium and then differentiated for 14 days to mature adipocytes before the start of the experiments.

Induction medium contained dexamethasone, insulin, ciglitazone, transferrin, biotin, and antibiotics. 3- isobutyl-1-methylxanthine (IBMX) was added for the first 48 hours of differentiation; then was removed. Medium was changed every 2 days. The appearance of lipid inclusions was confirmed by adding Oil Red-O (AnaSpec, San Jose, California).

Test solutions were mixed 1:1 with media after appropriate dilutions were determined by a dose–response experiment. Solutions were placed on the cells for 12 hours, and the solution and substrate were rinsed before measuring glycerol, triglycerides, and lactate dehydrogenase in the medium. Oil Red-O staining of lipid in remaining cells allowed additional means of quantifying cell lysis (**Fig. 3**).

Four assays were planned: lactate dehydrogenase and Oil Red-O, both to test cytotoxicity, and glycerol and triglyceride, which specifically test for lipolysis (**Table 1**). The lactate dehydrogenase assay is a nonspecific cell death indicator. It defines the cytotoxicity of a substance. The Oil Red-O assay is a test in which the cells that remain are stained, and the surface and volume of the remaining living cells are measured in order to determine the degree of cytotoxicity caused by each test solution.

The glycerol assay specifically measures lipolysis. Glycerol, a product of fat hydrolysis, was quantified in this assay. The triglyceride assay is also specific for lipolysis. This independent study confirms that deoxycholate alone is the formula element that induces cell death. Phosphatidylcholine, when combined with an inert solvent, causes no adipocyte lysis. Other constituent ingredients

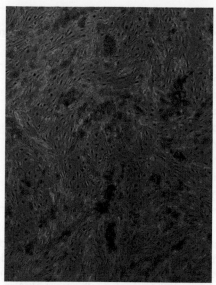

Fig. 3. Human adult derived adipocytes stained with Oil Red-O.

thought to have a lipolytic effect, benzyl alcohol and Isuprel, caused no adipocyte lysis in any of the four assays.

There is a clear difference in the effect of more concentrated versus more dilute deoxycholate, as demonstrated by **Fig. 4**. The elements that read 100 show the same adipolytic activity as the saline control: none. There is a significant, but not linear increase in the potency of deoxycholate with increasing concentration.

SAFETY AND EFFICACY OF INJECTION LIPOLYSIS IN *FELIS CATTUS*

The paucity of published animal studies is partly because of difficulty in finding a suitable animal for treatment. Rittes' study on rabbits[5] used the dorsal fat pad found in large female rabbits. Few animals have a subcutaneous fat distribution similar to that of people. To adhere to Animal Care and Use Committee (ACUC) protocol, only the least complex animal that would achieve the study goal would be approved for study use. Cats were chosen as the study animal, because their abdominal fat distribution is very similar to that of most humans—a thinner layer in the epigastrum, a moderate amount in the periumbilical region, and a much thicker fat pad in the suprapubic region.

In conjunction with Colorado State University, an approval of the ACUC-compliant, prospective double-blind randomized study protocol was granted using 12 fat cats as subjects. The purpose of the study was to test the safety and efficacy of

Table 1
Averaged results with all assays: lactate dehydrogenase, Oil Red-O glycerol, triglyceride

Test Solution	Adipocyte Cell Lysis Obtained with this Solution
PC50/ DC42	++
Deoxycholate 1%	+++
Deoxycholate 2.4%	+++
Phosphatidycholine 5% in mineral oil	0
Isuprel 0.08% injectable	0
Local anesthetic 5%	0
Saline 0.9% (control)	0
Benzyl alcohol	0

the standard PC50/DC42 formula, a modified PC/DC formula of slightly lesser strength in order to reduce adverse effects from phosphatidylcholine and deoxycholate, and a saline control. A second goal was to determine the value, if any, of more than one treatment session. The third parameter measured was the degree of skin retraction achieved following injection treatments. Overall efficacy of fat reduction was examined. Strict adherence to humane and gentle treatment of the subjects was followed. All cats were allowed free feeding, and could eat an unlimited quantity of food at any time.

Materials and Methods

Twelve cats were treated over a period of 4 months. Two different PC/DC-based formulas and a saline control were tested. The cats were divided into three groups. One group had a single injection session; the second group underwent two injection sessions, and the third group had three injection sessions before harvest of the treatment regions and subsequent closure.

All cats were weighed before each treatment session, and a standardized abdominal girth was measured. The abdominal fur was clipped closely, and inhalation anesthesia was induced. Sterile preparation of the abdomen was performed before each procedure. During the first treatment

session, all cats received a manual tattoo of three 38 mm circles in the abdominal midline (**Fig. 5**). One circle was placed in the epigastrum, one near the umbilicus, and the distal circle was located in the lower abdominal region. Caliper thickness of each fat pad was measured before any treatment using a small incision located at the inferior central base of all tattooed circles. Using a sterile marking pen, a grid was traced within each circle, with a 0.8 cm spacing of injection sites. A 0.1 cc dose of formula was injected in each demarcated spots using a 6 mm 27 gauge needle. A total of 13 injections or 1.3 cc of formula was injected per circle.

Because the formulas were randomized to maintain objectivity, the injection locations of formulas A, B, and C also were randomized, because of the variation in thickness of fat pads in the epigastric, periumbilical, and suprapubic sites. In group 1, the injection pattern was designated as ABC. That is, the epigastric circle was injected with formula A, the periumbilical with formula B, and the lower abdominal region was treated with formula C. Group 2 was designated as the BCA group, while group 3 was the CAB group.

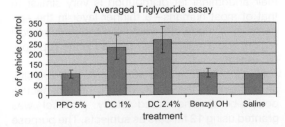

Fig. 4. Averaged triglyceride assay.

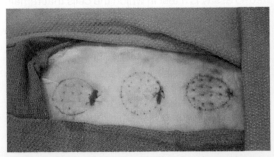

Fig. 5. Pattern of injections and fat pad thickness measurements.

The cats ranged in weight from 3.51 kg to 12.8 kg. To assure that some thinner and some fatter cats were included in all treatment groups, the cats were numbered according to increasing weight and girth, and cats 1, 4, 7, and 10 were treated with a single injection session. Cats 2, 5, 9, and 11 represented the two injection group, and the remaining cats received three injection sessions. Prior to each session, all animals were weighed and measured. At the time of tissue harvest, the caliper thickness of the fat pad again was measured. Closure of the harvested regions was performed using a vertically oriented bilateral skin flap advancement method.

The degree of feline skin retraction also was measured by tracing the tattooed circles before each subsequent treatment. The change in surface area was measured by employing the Miles method of surface area calculation.

Both gross anatomy and microscopic anatomy of each specimen were recorded. Histopathologic evaluation was provided by Loren Golitz, MD.

Results

All but two of the cats lost weight during the treatment period, despite the opportunity to eat at any time. Abdominal circumference remained the same for three of the smaller cats. In the nine cats that lost girth, a surprising mean of 6 cm were lost over the 3-month treatment duration. More injection sessions and a heavier starting weight were associated with more weight and girth loss, despite the free-feeding option. Mean weight before the study was 7.08 kg, and mean weight loss during the study was 0.75 kg. It is not clear if the formulas injected influenced the cats' appetite, or if the anesthesia or procedures created a decrease in food intake. The weight and girth loss would not be able to be explained by lipolysis alone, as the amount of fat necrosis seen following injection lipolysis was not massive.

The presence of palpable nodularity inside each of the tattooed circles was checked by two examiners before treatments 2, 3, and 4, when treatment regions were excised. At the conclusion of the study, the formula key noted that PC 50/ DC 42 was formula A; the saline control was formula B, and the light modified PC/DC formula was formula C. As expected, palpable nodules were noted in all circles treated with formula A and formula C. Most formula B circles exhibited no palpable nodules, but before the last procedure, slight nodularity was noted in the B circles in two of the four remaining cats. Although the palpable nodules measuring from 3 mm to 7 mm were noted once the treatment regions were removed from

regions A and C, the nodules in the two cats' B circles appeared to be very small regions of fibrous scarring, not fat necrosis.

The safety and efficacy of injection lipolysis in cats mirrored the human clinical experience. The cats tolerated the treatments well. Probably because skin characteristics are so different (fur-bearing versus bare skin), no real histamine response was seen in cats.

The cats were not treated with postinjection pain medication, as none exhibited any outward signs of discomfort in the treatment region. Daily checks of the treatment sites were performed. On day 10, one cat developed a small area of skin loss (1 cm^2) in the distal treatment region next to an old spay scar. The formula injected in the region was PC50/ DC42. The region healed quickly and was difficult to discern by day 14.

Gross anatomy was very similar to that of people. Although the cat fat appeared almost white in comparison to the yellow of human fat, the clinical grayish appearance of fat necrosis was very similar in both cats and people. The fractionated response—areas of fat necrosis with apparent normal tissue between injected regions—was similar in both species also. **Fig. 6** shows a segment of cat fat injected with PC50/ DC 42, 1 month previously. Note fat necrosis in the 12 o'clock and 7 o'clock positions.

Microscopic histologic evaluation of the cats' subcutaneous fat and skin showed a difference in the skin region caused by the presence of clumps of hair in the papillary dermis. No fat necrosis was

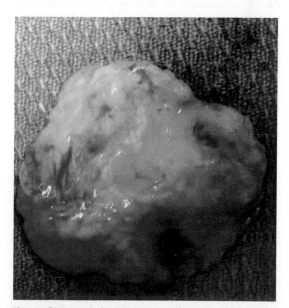

Fig. 6. Fat necrosis is seen in the 12 o'clock and 7 o'clock positions.

seen in the regions treated with saline injections. Regions treated with both PC50/DC42 (formula A) and half-strength PC/DC (formula C) showed focal fat necrosis at the injection sites. As expected, markers of fat necrosis included lysis of adipocyte cell walls, an infiltrate of polymorphonuclear leucocytes and lymphocytes, the presence of macrophages clearing cellular debris, angiogenesis, and the thickening of fibrous septae encasing fat globules. One characteristic present in cats that is not seen in people was the occasional presence of an unusual crystal formation in treated regions not seen in the human subjects.

The value of more than one treatment was clear. On gross examination, cats treated with a bioactive agent during one injection session had up to 13 visible nodules of fat necrosis.

The two-treatment fat pads had many more regions of fat necrosis, and the fat clinically appeared firmer. The three treatment fat pads were much more solid than those treated with a saline control or fewer injection sessions. Although the measurable fat pad thickness was not significantly changed by caliper measurement calculations, the flabby character of the tissue treated was changed into a more firm tissue type that held its shape when cut.

To measure skin retraction, or possible decrease of skin surface area in the treatment region, a 38 mm circle was tattooed using a surgical cookie cutter pattern around each treatment region. Prior to each treatment, each cats' treatment regions were traced onto a piece of clear acetate for later surface area measurement. At the conclusion of all treatments, the acetate patterns were weighed on an analytic balance having a capacity of 120 g, which reads to the 0.0001 g; linearity of about 0.0002 g; internal calibration three times. The median weight of each circle was compared with that of the control 38 mm acetate circle to determine the degree of expansion or reduction of skin surface area.

The results of these measurements showed no statistically significant change in skin surface area in the cats as a group. Some of the cats, however, had significant surface area reduction, especially in the thinner cats. It is hard to extrapolate these results to people, as cat skin is different from human skin in two respects. The obvious major difference is that the cat skin structure is fur-bearing, while most human skin has only a few hairs in comparison. The other difference is that in people, the dermal/fat junction is marked by peninsulas of fat poking up into the base of the dermis, and by small segments of dermis protruding into the underlying fat. The cats' dermal/fat junction is somewhat more uniform.

Summary

The one constant that was noted throughout the cat study was how localized the reaction to the injections was. No large confluent areas of fat necrosis were seen. The necrosis induced never appeared outside the tattooed treatment margin, or below a depth of 1.0 cm. Therefore, the deep fat in the distal treatment region remained untouched by injection lipolysis. The extent of fat necrosis overall was small, when gross specimens were evaluated. The message received from this strictly controlled study was that no large volumes of fat could be obliterated with this treatment; its best use is as a finesse superficial treatment for topographic contour correction.

MULTICENTER PROSPECTIVE CLINICAL STUDY

From July through October 2007, a multicenter clinical study evaluating the efficacy and safety of injection lipolysis in the back roll region was performed in Colorado and Virginia. A Clinical Review Organization (CRO)-reviewed protocol was followed, and all patients were screened for inclusion and exclusion criteria. All patient volunteers were interviewed, and a study consent was obtained before inception of the study.

Materials and Methods

Twenty patient volunteers began treatments, and 17 of the 20 completed all segments of the study. The region of the back roll bulging below the bra line was the targeted treatment region. Two injection sessions 4 weeks apart were planned. Inclusion criteria of a BMI of 28 or less, females between the ages of 28 and 60 in good health with no serious chronic disease, and no patients who were pregnant or breast feeding were strictly enforced. No patient who had an open sore in the treatment region, a soy allergy or sensitivity, or scleroderma or systemic lupus was included. Patients were instructed to avoid aspirin, ibuprofen, and other blood thinner-type products for the duration of the study.

The injection lipolysis solution combining phosphatidylcholine and sodium deoxycholate without a vasodilator was used (Masterpharm). Manual injections were used, with a 9 mm injection depth. The left and right back roll regions were treated. Pretreatment measurements of skin fold thickness from the base of the scapula to the linear depression at the base of the fat pad were performed. Preinjection history and physical examination preceded the first injection session. Standardized photographs were taken before each treatment session in the posteroanterior, oblique, and profile views. Before each treatment, the patient signed an informed consent. At the conclusion of the study, 6 weeks after the second injection session, measurements and photographs were repeated.

Each injection session was performed using a strict and reproducible format. The treatment region was circled with a surgical marker, and visual confirmation of the trouble spot by the patient was given. The marked treatment region was photographed. The most prominent protrusive ridge was marked, and injection points 1.5 cm apart were delineated. A slightly higher dose of 0.6 cc PC/DC would be injected in the region where the fat pad was thickest. The remaining surface area was gridded with a 1.5 cm pattern. 0.5 cc of PC/DC was injected in these regions, following sterile prep with chlorhexidine. The depth of injection was 9 mm. All regions were cleansed after completion of the injections, and a soft dressing was applied for 30 minutes.

All patients were examined at day 3 after injection, and immediately before the second injection session. A recheck at 3 days was performed following the second injection session also. Final photographs, measurements, and a satisfaction survey were performed at 6 weeks.

Results

All patients expressed a high rate of satisfaction in the outcome; a mean of 4.48 out of 5 (see **Box 1** for the scale used). Skin caliper thickness averaged 4.43 cm in the back roll region before treatment. At the conclusion of the study, mean skin caliper measurement was 4.21 cm. More evident than a measurable decrease in skin fold thickness was the flattening of the back roll bulge, and the correction of the apparent overhang. Neither of these changes was measurable except by photographic evaluation and patient comments.

Two patients felt that the procedure was uncomfortable enough that, despite the good results, they might decline to have it done again. One patient had mild postinjection nausea. All had palpable nodules in the treatment region at

3 weeks after injection. None had prolonged swelling or bruising, and no patients experienced skin loss, hyperpigmentation, secondary hypersensitivity, or a less than expected aesthetic result. Photographic results are shown in **Figs. 7–9**.

DISCUSSION

These studies confirmed some beliefs (**Box 2**) regarding injection lipolysis while also dispelling some myths (**Box 3**).

Clearly, the detergent effect proposed by Rotunda[17] is the mechanism of inducing adipocyte necrosis. Pathologic evaluation by two independent pathologists characterizes this reaction as toxic chemical necrosis. (R. Colby, personal communication, 2007).[21]

Dispersion or spread of the solution in the injected treatment region has been questioned.[22] This study and those demonstrated in a previous treatise[23] show that precise placement of the injections is critical to the final outcome. If there is too much distance between injection points, bulges caused by untreated skip areas will occur. The location of the tip of the injection needle is of paramount importance.

If the needle is intradermal, immediate skin loss may occur. Volume injected clearly affects the amount of fat that will undergo necrosis. There has been no documentation of the supposition that the injected solution will spread into underlying fascia or muscle. Histology supports a radial spread of less than 1 cm from the central injection point with up to 0.8 cc of injected solution at that point.

The role of phosphatidylcholine in injection lipolysis has been debated.[24–26] The studies presented here show three mechanisms of action of phosphatidylcholine. Given the pH of phosphatidylcholine is 7.0, and the pH of deoxycholate is 8.08 (S. Laddy, personal communication, 2008), one clear role of phosphatidylcholine is that of a buffer. Optimal human systemic pH is 7.4. The spread of the solution through the target tissue is not just mechanical; it also is affected by the degree of cytotoxicity exhibited by the solution. For example, plain sodium deoxycholate at a strength of 4.2%, or 42 mg/mL, will cause immediate fat necrosis in the region of injection. Therefore, the clinical result of using this formula will be dramatic and very localized fat necrosis without much dispersion.

The addition of phosphatidylcholine to deoxycholate not only buffers the reaction; phosphatidylcholine also acts a drug delivery system for deoxycholate by forming a noncovalent bond with deoxycholate and allowing the temporarily inactivated detergent to diffuse beyond the injection site. Phosphatidylcholine also is used for this

Box 1
Grading scale for satisfaction with treatment outcome

1 = Unsatisfactory; would not recommend
2 = Less than expected improvement
3 = Modest visible change
4 = Definite improvement
5 = Dramatic improvement, would recommend
    without reservation

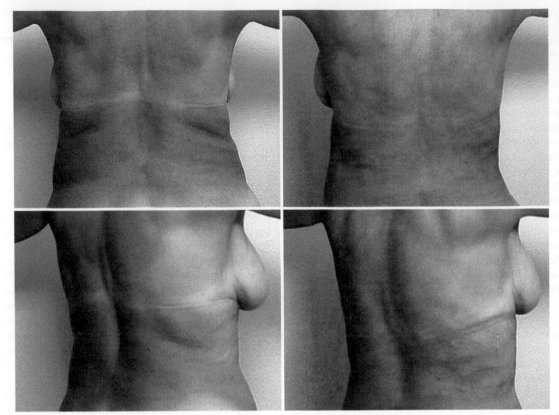

Fig. 7. 52-year-old patient is shown before *(upper and lower left)* and 4 weeks after *(upper and lower right)* two injection sessions in the back roll region. Note visible nodularity still present in the lower right photo. These nodules disappeared 1 month later.

drug delivery purpose in the chemotherapeutic drug Doxin.[27]

A third role of phosphatidylcholine in injection lipolysis appears to be that of a governor of the reaction. When added to deoxycholate, phosphatidylcholine reduces the intensity of the degree of fat necrosis and delays the entire process, causes a fractionation of the response, and thus reduces the formation of fibrous scar tissue produced by treatments with deoxycholate alone. Viable islands of adipocytes are seen in regions treated with PC/ DC 1 month after injection, while subcutaneous fat treated with DC alone exhibits massive fat necrosis with fibrosis. The use of plain deoxycholate for treating small, multiple lipomas works well, as the goal of treatment is eradication of all of the fat in the treatment region.

The use of unbuffered deoxycholate, however, might not create the optimal result when used to treat more superficial fat for cosmetic purposes. Reports of severe fibrosis causing restriction of range of motion, prolonged pain after injection, and intense inflammation, numbness, and a feeling of "skin like cobblestone cardboard" following enthusiastic treatments with deoxycholate alone should be taken into account before a practitioner considers treating large regions with this compound.

The effect of this knowledge on clinical applications is important. Injection lipolysis is much better used as a finesse procedure for topographic contour correction than for reducing large volumes of fat, or

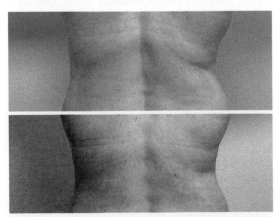

Fig. 8. 43-year-old patient with an asymmetric back roll is shown before *(above)* and 6 weeks after *(below)* two treatments with injection lipolysis.

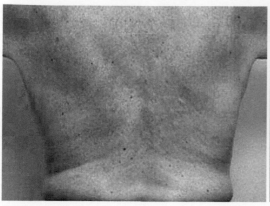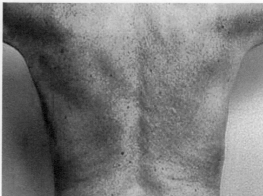

Fig. 9. 54-year-old patient is shown before *(left)* and after *(right)* two injection sessions with PC/DC in the back roll region.

for trying to tighten anything more than a mild skin laxity. Treatment goals should include preservation of soft tissue that easily glides over underlying muscle and bone. If a large amount of fibrous scar is produced with any treatment, whether it is aggressive liposuction or intense fat necrosis, there will be little or no soft tissue left in the subcutaneous layer. The skin will not glide over underlying structures. In severe cases, puckering or divots may be seen with motion in the treatment region.

Inappropriate recommendation for treatment of localized areas of excess fat may occur when the care provider has a limited number of treatment options. Examples of appropriate situations in which injection lipolysis could be reasonably recommended include: a patient who has residual bulges and divots following moderate liposuction, a swimsuit model who cannot get work because her inner thighs touch, an adult who has a thick fatty neck but no real skin excess, and a patient who has mild-to-moderate jowl formation.

Situations in which injection lipolysis should not be recommended include treatment of a patient who has a BMI over 30 who desires a reduction of abdominal fat, a young adult male who has firm, fibrous flank adiposity, an older chronically ill patient who has multiple regions of fatty excess and is trying to avoid surgery, and a patient who read on the Internet how injection lipolysis can eradicate unwanted fat without surgery.

Three histologic changes in the dermis overlying the treatment suggest mechanisms by which the clinically observed mild degree of skin retraction can be explained. The necrosis and subsequent obliteration of the peninsulas of fat protruding into the deep basal layer of the dermis appear to cause an accordion-like effect, drawing the basal dermis together. Another proposed mechanism for the generation of mild skin retraction is that of immediate subdermal inflammation. Histopathology shows angiogenesis in the subdermal fat and within the overlying dermis. Although it is probable that all three proposed mechanisms contribute to mild skin retraction and an improved appearance, none has been proven.

Fat necrosis, when examined histologically, has the following elements: visible disruption of the cell

> **Box 2**
> **Confirmed beliefs**
>
> Sodium deoxycholate is the cause of adipocyte lysis.
>
> The injection lipolysis solution disperses only locally, based on the mechanics of injection, depth of injection, formula used, spacing between injection sites, and the volume of solution injected.
>
> Phosphatidylcholine acts as a buffer to delay and diminish the dramatic effect of unopposed deoxycholate.
>
> Too much deoxycholate in the formula causes massive fat necrosis and changes in the skin overlying the treatment region.
>
> Injection lipolysis should be used as a finesse procedure, not for treating large volumes of excess subcutaneous fat.
>
> Three mechanisms of skin retraction in people are shown: diffuse intradermal inflammation in the skin overlying the treatment region, angiogenesis in the treatment region, and focal ablation of the fatty peninsulas extending up into the basal layer of the dermis.
>
> Fat necrosis similar to that seen in panniculitis, liposuction, and traumatic fat necrosis has been documented histologically. There is not a novel mechanism of action in injection lipolysis that will elevate liver enzymes or cause systemic damage beyond the treatment region.

Box 3
Myths dispelled

Apoptosis is the mechanism of action in injection lipolysis.

Phosphatidylcholine adds nothing to the injection lipolysis formula.

Patients can lose three dress sizes when treated with lipodissolve. The process can correct only small, well localized regions of soft fat.

There is no scientific basis proving that injection lipolysis works. Many well-designed studies are currently present in the literature substantiating the efficacy of this treatment modality.

---

membrane, inflammation, neovascularization, and macrophage infiltration to process the cellular debris. All of these elements are repeatedly present in 238 histology slides evaluated following injection lipolysis treatments. Studies performed immediately following injections[28,29] show no elevation in liver enzymes and no indications of any systemic effect of PC/DC. A frequent question by patients and the media is "where does the dead fat go?" No radionuclide studies tracing fat from the treatment region to another region appear available in the current literature.

Although most medical practitioners assume that necrotic fat and other tissue processed by macrophages undergoes beta oxidation in the liver, no hard scientific data confirm that the necrotic fat following liposuction, injection lipolysis, panniculitis, or traumatic fat necrosis follows that path. Currently no FDA-approved drug exists for injections in subcutaneous tissue to reduce fat. Although the FDA is investigating new drugs, it is incorrect to tell patients that the procedure and drugs are FDA-approved.

Another myth promoted by some injectors is that the FDA does not regulate PC/DC, as it is a food supplement. The metabolic and endocrine division of the FDA cites the original Food, Drug, and Cosmetic Act: "A substance is a drug if it is injected with the purpose of altering the structure or function of an animal or human." (P. Madara, personal communication, 2006)

Some injectors quote the "GRAS" rule, or "generally regarded as safe." Tradition within the medical community claims that a drug can be used in another pharmaceutical if it is contained in an FDA-approved formulation. In order for that rule to be applicable, the constituent ingredient in question must be used in the same or lesser concentration in the new formulation as it is present in the approved substance. Another erroneous claim is that PC/DC is being used off label. There would have to be an on label FDA-approved use for injectable PC/DC. Although Lipostabil (Aventis) is approved in Germany for intravenous injection to reduce coronary artery plaque, there is no FDA-approved use for PC/DC in the United States.

If the compound is not FDA-approved, how can it be legal to inject? In most states, the state board of pharmacy and state board of medicine regulates the practice of compounding. The rules for prescribing a compounded drug are strict, and have been clarified by the FDA recently. To comply with regulations, a physician must evaluate the patient and perform a history and physical evaluation. A recommendation for treatment with injection lipolysis would need to be documented, showing why commonly practiced alternatives are unsuitable. A prescription specifically for that patient only must be sent to the pharmacy, signed by the physician. These steps were taken to protect the patient and to minimize the practice of injection lipolysis by paramedical nonphysician practitioners. The patient should not be treated on the day of evaluation, and should review and sign a thorough, detailed informed consent before any treatment is given. Obtaining malpractice insurance covering for this treatment modality can be difficult. Although Doctors' company, which covers many plastic surgeons, offers coverage for those surgeons adhering to the standard of practice, many other insurance companies will not cover injecting physicians automatically. It is wise to check on the terms of coverage before adopting injection lipolysis into practice.

SUMMARY

Patient expectations define efficacy. Injection lipolysis should not be used when treating patients who have large volumes of fat, or patients who have unrealistic expectations. Injection lipolysis is a complement to liposuction and dermolipectomy in that it is a technique that can be used when neither of the other procedures will achieve the goals of treatment, when used as a finesse procedure, in regions with soft fat and mild skin retraction. Careful patient selection is critical, and if any doubt about the wisdom of using injection lipolysis exists, it should be avoided.

A truthful representation of the risks and benefits, advantages, and limitations of injection lipolysis will help the practitioner and the patient decide which procedure would suit him or her best.

REFERENCES

1. LeCoz J. Traite de mesotherapie. Paris: Masson; 2004.

2. Duncan DI, Hasengschwandtner F. Lipodissolve for subcutaneous fat reduction and skin retraction. Aesthet Surg J 2005;25:530–43.
3. Duncan DI, Chubaty R. Clinical safety data and standards of practice for injection lipolysis: a retrospective study. Aesthet Surg J 2006;26:575–85.
4. Rittes P. The use of phosphatidylcholine for correction of localized fat deposits. Aesthetic Plast Surg 2003;27(4):315–8.
5. Rittes P. Injection of phosphatidylcholine in fat tissue: experimental study of local action in rabbits. Aesthetic Plast Surg 2006;30(4):474–8.
6. Katocs A, Largis E, Allen D, et al. Perifused fat cells: effect of lipolytic agents. Available at: http://www.jbc.org/cgi/content/abstract/248/14/5089. Accessed February 2, 2008.
7. Available at: http://www.collegesportsscholarships.com/lose-weight-diet.htm. Accessed May 23, 2008.
8. Available at: http://www.firstpagefitness.com/love handler.html. Accessed April 18, 2008.
9. Thermo Fisher Scientific. Thermo scientific pierce cell lysis technical handbook. 2008.
10. Available at: http://www.sigmaaldrich.com.
11. Available at: http://www.chemistry.co.nz/detergent_class.htm. Accessed March 7, 2008.
12. Hasengschwandtner F. Phosphatidylcholine treatment to induce lipolysis. J Cosmet Dermatol 2005;4:308–13.
13. Peckitt N. Evidence-based practice. Yorkshire (UK): Jeremy Mills Publishing; 2005.
14. Palmer M, Curran J, Bowler P. Clinical experience and safety using phosphatidylcholine injections for the localized reduction of subcutaneous fat: a multi-centre, retrospective UK study. J Cosmet Dermatol 2006;5:218–26.
15. Rotunda AR, Kolodney MS. Mesotherapy and phosphatidycholine injections: historical clarification and review. Dermatol Surg 2006;32(4):465–80.
16. Rose PT, Morgan M. Histological changes associated with mesotherapy for fat dissolution. J Cosmet Laser Ther 2005;7:17–9.
17. Rotunda AR, Suzuki H, Moy RL, et al. Detergent effects of sodium deoxycholate are a major feature of an injectable phosphatidylcholine formulation used for localized fat dissolution. Dermatol Surg 2004;30:1001–8.
18. Hasengschwandtner F. Injection lipolysis for effective reduction of localized fat in the place of minor lipoplasty. Aesthet Surg J 2006;26:125–30.
19. Available at: http://www.freepatentsonline.com. Patent # 20050267080.
20. Pharmaceuticals initiate phase II study of its adipolytic agent for reduction of submental fat. Available at: http://www.kytherabiopharma.com. Accessed January 10, 2008.
21. Golitz L. Presented at: Dermatopathology conference. Denver, July 27, 2008.
22. The American Society of Aesthetic Plastic Surgery. Fat-melting fad: too good to be true?. Available at: http://www.surgery.org./press/news-release.
23. Duncan DI, Palmer M. Fat reduction using phosphatidylcholine/sodium deoxycholate injections: standard of practice. Aesthetic Plast Surg 2008;32(6):858–72.
24. Motolese P. Phospholipids do not have lipolytic activity: a critical review. J Cosmet Laser Thor 2008;10(2):114–8.
25. Hasengschwandtner F. Injection lipolysis basics. Presented at: First International Convention for Lipodissolve. Salzburg, Austria, 18 2005.
26. Rotunda A. Overview of mesotherapy and injection lipolysis. Presented at: International Mesolipotherapy instructional course. Las Vegas, 2006.
27. Formarie T. Doxorubicin biocompatible O/W microemulsion stabilized by mixed surfactant colloids containing soya phosphatidylcholine. Colloids Surf B Biointerfaces 2006;51(1):54–61.
28. Hexsel D, Orlandi C, Zeichmeister do Prado D. Cosmetic use of injectable phosphatidylcholine on the face. Otolaryngol Clin North Am 2005;38:1119–29.
29. Meissner C. Complications with lipodissolve. Presented at: First International Convention for Lipodissolve. Salzburg, Austria, July 18, 2005.

Comment on "Refinement of Technique in Injection Lipolysis Based on Scientific Studies and Clinical Evaluation"

Juarez M. Avelar, MD

"Refinement of Technique in Injection Lipolysis Based on Scientific Studies and Clinical Evaluation," by Dr. Diane Duncan and colleagues, presents a very clear and didactic description of injection lipolysis with accurate clinical evaluation for treatment and behavior of fat cells after injection. Studies, concepts, and clinical evaluations demonstrate that injection lipolysis is a good and useful procedure to remove small areas of localized adiposities beneath the skin. The authors demonstrate scientifically by microscopy studies that fat cells are damaged by subcutaneous fat injected with deoxycholate. It is well known that after fat necrosis the adipose tissue does not regenerate. This is a useful step to reduce the number of fat cells of localized adiposities. This scientific article discusses nonsurgical fat reduction caused by adiposity lysis or fat necrosis.

The authors also injected a formula consisting of a combination of phosphatidylcholine and sodium deoxycholate, producing thickening of fibrous septae and fat necrosis. These alterations on the subcutaneous layers were demonstrated scientifically to reduce localized adiposities after treatment with injection lipolysis. Good results were seen in 17 of the 20 volunteer patients who underwent injection of lipolysis. Duncan and colleagues found that all patients were pleased with the treatment, did not complain about the procedure, and had a high rate of satisfaction. The patients presented in the article were treated with injections on regions of the back with localized adiposities.

Furthermore, the authors studied the reaction and behavior of the subcutaneous tissue on cats and found local reaction of fat necrosis. They also demonstrated that reaction was well localized without confluent areas of fat necrosis. Even the deep fat was not damaged, which means that the effects of injection lipolysis remain superficially on the same level.

Regarding treatment by lipolysis, body contouring surgery has greatly improved since 1977 when Illouz presented at the French Society[1] a liposuction technique that became popularized after 1981.[2] The surgical principles described by Illouz were to inject hypotonic solution before the operation to produce hydrotomy, followed by suction of the fat. In his first descriptions and presentations he emphasized the importance of lipolysis during the liposuction operation. Today, his method has become one of the most important procedures performed by plastic surgeons all over the world. Liposuction technique is a very useful contribution for removing localized adiposities to treat most abnormalities of the human body to improve body contour.

In addition to the importance of liposuction as a surgical technique itself, it can be used in combination with traditional methods, which has opened a wide field in plastic surgery. To understand such combined procedures, the treatment of several abnormalities of the abdominal wall, selection of patients is a mandatory step for indication of the surgical technique before operation.[3] Abdominoplasty combined with liposuction has become a standard operation because several deformities may be treated simultaneously: localized adiposities, resection of excess skin, and reinforcement of the rectus abdominalis caused by flaccidity of

E-mail address: juarez.m.avelar@uol.com.br

Clin Plastic Surg 36 (2009) 211–213
doi:10.1016/j.cps.2008.11.011
0094-1298/08/$ – see front matter © 2009 Published by Elsevier Inc.

the muscles and diastases. Several other regions of the body, such as the upper extremities, medial thigh, flanks, and torso, may also be treated through combined procedures of liposuction with panniculus resection using traditional methods. Those procedures are very useful for removing localized adiposities in the deeper layer of the panniculus, below the superficial fascia.[4,5]

Nevertheless, superficial liposuction is an important approach to remove localized adiposities from the areolar layer, which is above the superficial fascia, to reshape the surface of the body. That procedure, which was introduced and well described by Toledo[6,7] and Gasparotti,[8] is particularly indicated to treat the regions where the areolar layer may be thicker than the lamellar layer, such as the torso, upper abdomen, submental and submandibular areas, and the upper and lower extremities.[4] It should be emphasized, however, that the basal layer of the dermis must be preserved during every surgical procedure to avoid any damage to the skin. Damage to that layer may result in the development of severe irregularities to the cutaneous structures, which give ungraceful and unaesthetic results. Through use of the Toledo V-tip cannula it is possible to perform dissection, aspiration, and injection of fat, which may provide outstanding surgical results.

People the world over are always looking for a new treatment to lose weight, to have a better shape, and to improve body contour. There are millions of people, however, who do not care about beauty or expect a better body shape and are overweight or even morbidly obese. Such problems need clinical treatment with several kinds of drugs prescribed by a physician to achieve an adequate result. These patients also need well-balanced diets elaborated by outstanding nutritionists to achieve satisfactory results, but in most cases diet alone is not enough.

Nevertheless, millions of patients take drugs without medical care despite the risks to themselves. In addition to the use of unknown drugs, the public may accept several nonsurgical fat reduction treatments, hoping to improve their body contour. There are also local treatments known as "mesotherapy," which when it is well performed may reduce the volume of fat cells in localized adiposities. Those procedures, called "intradermal therapy," do not reduce the number of adipose cells; instead, they try to evacuate the fat from inside each unit of fat tissue.

Every day there are new machines shown on television, in newspapers and magazines, and on the Internet, which are the result of industry trying to sell fantasy and a miracle to the public. That sort of commercial business is more and more popular all over the world. There are external procedures performed by outstanding surgeons, however, which may treat properly localized adiposity with excellent results.

Concerning the current state of nutrition, humankind presents with two opposite situations: there is not enough food for the entire population of the world, and a very high percentage of the world population presents with diseases secondary to excessive ingestion of food. Unfortunately, medicine and the physician are between both situations. Medicine must give some support to the governments of poor countries to enable them to provide more food to their populations. Physicians of several specialties, even laboratories, have to work hard researching new drugs to treat diseases resulting from excessive food consumption.

Besides the constant effort to find new treatment, many patients need specific operations (eg, bariatric surgeries) and afterward resection of excessive panniculus on several regions of the body because of massive weight lost. All of the problems resulting from excessive ingestion of food or endocrine disturbances are a constant challenge for doctors.

Duncan and colleagues state that the purpose of their article is to describe scientifically the efficiency of the use of phosphatidylcholine and sodium deoxycholate, which produce adipose lysis to treat small areas of superficial localized adiposities. Previous publications already showed the efficiency of this method for correction of localized fat deposits. The authors present a very interesting article with excellent illustrations that is an outstanding contribution to body contour remodeling operations. The reaction and behavior of fat are shown in excellent microscopic photos after injections in both humans and cats. Such procedures are well indicated to reduce areas of localized adiposities and also to correct remaining local adiposities or irregularities after liposuction.

REFERENCES

1. Illouz YG. Une nouvelle technique pour les lipodystrophies localisées. La Revue de Chirurgie Esthétique de Langue Française 1980;6(19):10–2.
2. Illouz YG. Body contouring by lipolysys: a 5 year experience with over 3000 cases. Plast Reconstr Surg 1983;72(5):591.
3. Avelar JM. Fat-suction versus abdominoplasty. Aesthetic Plast Surg 1985;9:265–76.
4. Avelar JM. Regional distribution and behavior of the subcutaneous tissue concerning selection and indication for liposuction. Aesthetic Plast Surg 1989;13: 155–65.

5. Avelar JM. Abdominoplasty: new concepts for a new technique. Presented at the XXVI Annual International Symposium of Aesthetic Plastic surgery, Puerto Vallarta, Jalisco, Mexico, November 12 to 16, 1999.

6. Toledo LS. Total liposculpture. In: Gasparotti M, Lewis CM, Toledo LS, editors. Superficial liposculpture. New York: Springer-Verlag; 1993. p. 44.

7. Toledo LS, Mauad R. Complications of body sculpture: prevention and treatment. Clin Plast Surg 2006; 33:1–11.

8. Gaparotti M. Superficial liposuction: a new application of the technique for aged and flaccid skin. Aesthetic Plast Surg 1992;16(2):141–53.

The Lipodissolve Technique: Clinical Experience

Patrícia Guedes Rittes, MD

KEYWORDS

- Fat • Adipose tissue • Aging
- Lipodissolve • Phosphatidylcholine

The performance of different treatments in the field of cosmiatry and of continuous research to clarify and improve well-known and newer techniques has shown that, although they were designed primarily to treat several conditions, the lipodissolve technique and mesotherapy should be seen as specific tools for specific purposes, that is, as appropriate treatments for specific symptoms. As such, it is important to emphasize the difference between lipodissolve and mesotherapy. Although both techniques involve injections, they are distinguished by definition in their respective uses in improving face and body contouring, skin elasticity, and fat melting.

Mesotherapy, the treatment of the skin's middle layers, is a specialized medical treatment created in France in 1953 by Dr. Michel Pistor who successfully applied it to patients with a variety of medical conditions. Mesotherapy entails injections of various vitamins, minerals, and amino acids into the skin and is primarily intended to treat some injuries, skin conditions, and cellulite. The procedure consists of local administration of selected medications to promote skin rejuvenation, glow, and turgor and to prevent it. Since Dr. Pistor developed mesotherapy, it has been applied by thousands of physicians all over the world and is a powerful tool in the treatment of many medical and aesthetic conditions.

Since the introduction of lipodissolve in 1995 in São Paulo, Brazil, and the establishment of protocols and parameters for its use, research on this technique has continued. Lipodissolve is a nonsurgical treatment to reduce fat deposits via the injection of a single component, phosphatidylcholine,

a natural product found in the body. The main role of phosphatidylcholine in the body is to help emulsify and break down fat and cholesterol; it is a key constituent of cell membranes and high-density lipoproteins. The phosphatidylcholine used in lipodissolution is derived from soybeans and has the same molecular structure as phosphatidylcholine in the body.

Research on the role of phosphatidylcholine in reducing or eliminating fatty deposits in the body has demonstrated that its main compound, lecithin, is a natural mixture of the diglycerides of stearic, palmitic, and oleic acids linked to the choline group of phosphoric acid. The compound is commonly referred to as PPC and is found naturally in living plants and animals. Polyunsaturated PPC is a standardized and highly purified soybean lecithin extract that has been used orally in the treatment and prophylaxis of arteriosclerosis, hyperlipidemia, hepatitis, fat embolism, diabetes, and hypercholesterolemia since the 1960s. In addition, soy lecithin functions as a surfactant, emulsifier, and skin-conditioning agent. Data on product formulation that were submitted to the US Food and Drug Administration (FDA) in 1997 indicated that lecithin was an ingredient found in 674 cosmetic products. Moreover, the systemic safety and efficacy of PPC and other natural phospholipids as blood lipid–lowering drugs has been well described.

When I first injected Lipostabil Endovena (Nattermann & Cie, Köln, Germany) (ie, PPC 250 mg/5 mL) directly into fat deposits, I believed its action would help break down and emulsify the fat deposits as it used the body's natural methods

Santa Casa de Misericórdia Medical School, São Paulo, Brazil
E-mail address: prittes@terra.com.br

Clin Plastic Surg 36 (2009) 215–221
doi:10.1016/j.cps.2008.11.003
0094-1298/08/$ – see front matter © 2009 Published by Elsevier Inc.

of excreting fat to permanently reduce fat deposits. One end of the molecule of phosphatidylcholine is hydrophilic and the other lipophilic, acting on bile acids. Several other studies have shown that deoxycolate (DC) is the major emulsifying feature that causes the necrosis of fatty cells, and PPC works as a tampon solution and decreases the aggressive action of DC.

After injection, the Lipostabil formula from Aventis (Sanofi-Aventis U.S., Bridgewater, New Jersey), which is phosphatidylcholine plus deoxycholate (PPC/DC), a detergent, breaks down the structure of the fat cell, provoking an intense inflammatory process and necrosis of the cell. This formula of PPC/DC (Lipostabil) is especially effective in treating problem fat areas that may not be eliminated with diet and exercise alone. It has been used for reducing fat deposits for about 12 years but has been used for other medical purposes for much longer. Since 1959, it has been used intravenously to dissolve atheromatosis plaques in cardiac disease.

Lipodissolve is a relatively new aesthetic procedure used to dissolve smallish, localized, and defined zones of fat in the face and body. The injections exclusively contain Lipostabil, with PPC/DC as the fat-emulsifying substance. In Brazil, the technique was pioneered by the author in 1995 complying with established standards and protocols. Lipolysis consists of injecting larger quantities, when compared with mesotherapy, subcutaneously at a depth of approximately 12 mm into the fat tissue. Results have been very good. Completely natural, the injections produce no adverse effects and no threat to overall health.

HISTORY AND CLINICAL EXPERIENCE

Lipodissolve was first presented at the 54th Brazilian Dermatology Congress in Belo Horizonte, Brazil, in September 1999 as a "Correction of Lower Lid Bulging by Using Phosphatidylcholine." The lipodissolving technique originated when several patients asked for a way to improve their tired-looking eyes without undergoing the traditional blepharoplasty surgery. These patients presented with prominent periorbital fat pads, often having a persistent tired look. The objective in these cases was to develop a nonsurgical treatment of the fat pads. The first patient was treated with excellent results, and, subsequently, 30 patients were treated with phosphatidylcholine injections for prominent lower eyelid fat pads.

Pre- and posttreatment photographs were taken for long-term analysis. A marked reduction of the lower eyelid fat pads was noted over the 2-year follow-up period with no recurrences. It was concluded that the injection of phosphatidylcholine (250 mg/5 mL) into the fat pads is a simple office procedure that may postpone or even substitute for lower eyelid blepharoplasty.

The physiology of the change in the eyelids involves herniation of the infraorbital fat pads, resulting in a prominence of the lower eyelids causing patients to have a tired and aged appearance. These deformities consist of skin, subcutaneous fat, orbicular muscle, and suborbicular fat. Orbital fat exerts pressure on the septum and the orbicular muscle, causing a bulge. What appears to be excess skin is often merely the herniation caused by the fat pad appearing under the skin. This deformity is classically managed by surgical resection or reinsertion of the herniated fat into the orbital cavity, and the continuous suture of the capsular palpebral fascia maintains it in its original position.

The author's study followed the guidelines of the 1975 Declaration of Helsinki. An informed consent form was obtained from all individuals. Preoperative evaluation included examining the size and location of fat pads. Photographs were obtained and coexisting ocular pathology checked. Varying degrees of bulge in the fat pads were treated. The 50 patients ranged in age from 30 to 70 years.

The procedure was performed in an outpatient setting with the patient seated. The skin of the lower lid was pulled downward with the forefinger, and gentle pressure was applied over the globe for visualization of the fat pad. Pure phosphatidylcholine (0.4 mL; 250 mg/5 mL) was injected into the infraorbital fat pad by using a 0.5-in, 30-gauge needle and distributed among the bulging periorbital fat pads (central, medial, and lateral), based on the individual patient's need. Injections were given at 15-day intervals to allow complete resolution of infraorbital swelling. Five patients were given a total of three applications, 12 patients a total of two applications, and 11 patients a total of one application.

Common and expected reactions to the treatment included immediate edema, erythema, and a mild burning sensation that resolved within a half hour. Edema of the entire lower lid was noted over the initial 6 hours and persisted up to 72 hours. This reactive inflammatory process that occurs after the shot leads to fibrosis and causes the retraction of the skin at the end of the treatment period. All of the patients reported dramatic improvement of their eyelid bulges. There were no complications, hematomas, allergic reactions, infections, or skin contour irregularities.

The earliest English-language article describing the aesthetic use of phosphatidylcholine was published in 2001,[1–4] reporting on the research and initial experience with the technique. Until then, the treatment of this deformity was surgical. Lipodissolve offered a noninvasive, office-based procedure.

After the eye pads had been treated with lipodissolution for many years, research on the technique developed a broader scope prompted by the good quality of the responses obtained and by a patient who did not want to under go liposuction due to the risks involved in surgery. In 1998 a famous television star in Brazil went into a coma during liposuction. The same formula and technique were used to treat localized fat deposits and obtained very good results. A report on this use of lipodissolution was published in 2003.[5–7] Reactions to this report were positive. In the study, small- to medium-sized unwanted fat deposits that were not reduced by diet or exercise were dissolved by lipodissolution. The earlier use of phosphatidylcholine provided a new technique of body contouring by dissolving small fat deposits that persisted after exercise or liposuction.

The most common areas treated with lipodissolution are abdominal bulges, "love handles," "saddle bags" on the thighs, buttocks, and arms. In men, it can be used to reduce chest fat. Before the treatment, patients are measured and pictures taken. The treatment area is then systematically injected with pure Lipostabil. A similar protocol of injections every 15 days has yielded satisfactory results without complications.

Through extensive research and application in Brazil, a specific technique for using PPC to dissolve body fat deposits has been developed. For body contouring, the total area to be injected is always the same. An area measuring 80 cm^2 is divided into six points, and 0.8 mL is injected at each point, approximately 2 cm apart. Symptoms of itching, burning, erythema, and edema typically remain for 48 hours. The procedure may be repeated at 2 weeks for a total of one to four sessions. Nodules and bruises may appear in the injected areas; however, they usually disappear spontaneously in 1 to 2 weeks. Sensitivity of the treated area may vary from one region to another. Compressive garments may aid in patient comfort, especially for the abdomen and legs. Bruises are to be expected and resolve naturally on their own.

A maximum of 10 mL (two Lipostabil 5-mL vials) is injected in the first dose. The physician should distribute the dose evenly in the 80 cm^2 area and observe the patient's reaction to the injections carefully. When treating multiple areas of the body during the same session, the physician may inject up to eight vials of 5 mL per session. The procedure may be repeated from one to four times, 2 weeks apart, followed by waiting 3 months to allow skin to retract.

Clinical experience has shown that most patients who undergo this treatment achieve their goals within four sessions; however, this requires that the patient maintain his or her body weight within a range that is close to the ideal. If the patient gains more than 4 kg, the effect of PPC injections will be lost.

The lipodissolve technique was so successful that physicians from several cities wanted to learn the procedure. Subsequently, the author conducted more than 300 workshops on all continents to certify professionals to use it. She has taught more than 1000 physicians to reproduce the technique in their offices and clinics.

The success of the lipodissolve technique brought to light the newest use of Lipostabil Endovena, which led to an increase in clinical research and experimental studies.[8–11] To better understand the mechanism of PPC, the author conducted an experimental study in rabbits that demonstrated that the fat injected with PPC was destroyed at the site. In addition, histopathologic studies on specimens showed that the action of PPC was localized and therefore safe.[8] A subsequent study was performed to determine any complications with the use of PPC, and the results indicated no adverse effects.[12]

During this study period, letters seeking information on adverse effects were sent to physicians in hospitals, medical schools, emergency rooms, and medical societies in Brazil and to workshop participants abroad. The purpose of the letters was to inquire about any case of complications or any report of harm caused by the subcutaneous use of phosphatidylcholine. None of the physicians reported adverse effects of using the technique.

Aging Neck

Treating a case of gynecomastia to lift masculine nipples led to the idea that if it were possible to lift nipples by fibrosis, the same result might be achieved in the aging neck and jaw line. The idea proved to be correct. A markedly younger looking jaw line can be achieved by injecting 0.3 mL into three points along the jaw line and 3 cm below it, causing a retraction of the skin and consequent improvement of its appearance. The results of this study have been submitted for publication (**Figs. 1–3**).

SUMMARY OF THE PROCEDURE

The following list indicates the steps physicians should use when performing lipodissolution:

- Determine full health conditions.
- Diagnose and ensure the patient's suitability for the treatment.

- Give detailed information on the procedure; clarify all doubts.
- Advise the patient of possible collateral effects inherent to the treatment.
- Have a consent form signed.
- Have the patient photographed.
- Seat the patient in comfortable position when treating the eye pads.
- Have body areas marked.
- Place the patient in a comfortable prone position when treating body areas if necessary.
- Prepare injections.
- Pinch skin and fat, never muscle.
- Inject solution.
- Observe the patient's reaction and wait for approximately 15 minutes.
- Give the patient take-home instructions as follows:

  Do not use a compress or ice pads.

  Do not touch the injected area.

  Wear sunglasses after treatment of eye pads.

  Use a pillow on the first night after treatment.

  Do not perform physical exercise.

  Edema and bruises resolve naturally.
- Repeat treatment at 15-day intervals for at most four sessions.
- If additional treatment is necessary, wait 3 months.

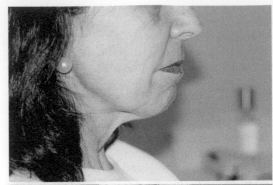

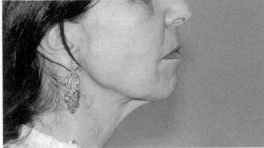

Fig. 2. A 56-year-old patient with an aging neck is shown before and after three sessions.

INDICATIONS

The lipodissolve technique has the following indications: (1) to treat tired eyes (ie, nonsurgical treatment of the fat pads and lower and upper eyelids); (2) to sculpt the body (ie, nonsurgical treatment of localized fat in the abdomen, thighs, arms, love handles, and buttocks); and (3) to address the aging neck with impressive improvement as the technique provokes a retraction of the skin.

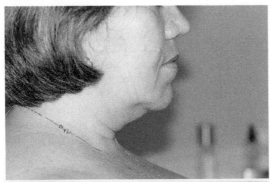

Fig. 1. A 48-year-old patient with an aging neck is shown before and after two sessions.

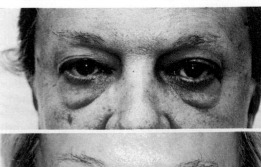

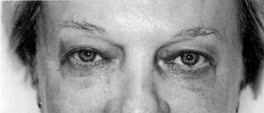

Fig. 3. A 51-year-old patient with fat pads is shown before and after four sessions.

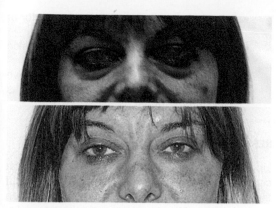

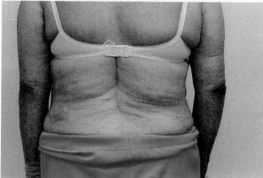

Fig. 4. A 37-year-old patient with fat pads is shown before and after six sessions.

CONTRAINDICATIONS

Lipodissolve is suitable only for patients who are seeking to reduce localized fat deposits that are resistant to dietary changes or exercise. It is not used primarily for weight reduction; rather, it is used for body sculpting.

Patients who are pregnant, breastfeeding, or planning on pregnancy in the next 6 months are not suitable for lipodissolve treatments. Persons less than 18 years of age and those with an alteration of blood clotting (hemophilia) are not candidates for lipodissolving treatments.

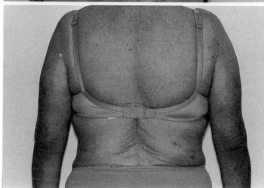

Fig. 6. A 57-year-old patient with local fat deposits due to chronic cortisone use is shown before and after 20 sessions.

CHOOSING A PATIENT

Choosing the appropriate patient is of extreme importance. The physician must be conservative

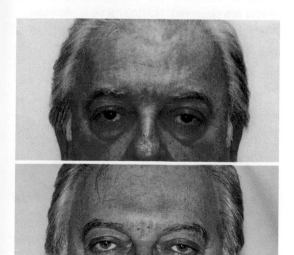

Fig. 5. A 55-year-old patient with fat pads is shown before and after two sessions.

and cautious, because this technique is not suitable for every patient or every condition involving localized fat. The technique helps treat some areas of localized fat, not obese patients. It is definitely not an overall "slimming" technique. Patients must be informed of all collateral effects, have all doubts addressed, and sign a consent form. Before and after photographs should be taken (**Figs. 4–6**).

A diagnosis of excess fat is essential, because PPC can only treat fat and not muscle, skin, or connective tissue.

TECHNIQUE OUTLINE
Fat Pads

The physician considering treatment of fat pads may find fat, muscle, connective tissue, and excess skin. To diagnose correctly, the physician needs to identify accurately whether the fat is essential, because PPC only treats fat. Before and after photographs must be taken. The procedure is performed as follows:

- Clean the skin.
- Inject 0.4 mL of PPC into each eye as follows:
  0.1mL in the lateral bulge

0.2mL in the medial bulge
0.1mL in the central bulge
- Repeat on the other eye.

Immediately after the injection, the patient experiences a mild burning, sticking, and heavy sensation that lasts for about 15 minutes and is followed by severe edema. This edema takes about 72 hours to resolve. No compresses, ice, or other procedure should be used. The PPC injections should be repeated from one to four times and generally take 3 months to attain total retraction of the skin. Reinjection should be performed again if necessary.

Body Fat Deposits

The physician should diagnose correctly. The procedure is performed as follows:

- Clean approximately 80 cm^2 of the skin and divide it into six points.
- Inject 0.8 mL in each point, approximately 2 cm apart.
- Itching, burning, and erythema remain for at most 20 minutes. Swelling remains for 72 hours. Bruises may occur but heal spontaneously. If nodules appear, do not inject them in the following session. They take 1 or 2 months to resolve naturally.

Sensitivity varies from one area to other, and compression may be indicated to minimize discomfort in the lower abdomen. A maximum dose of PPC, 10 mL, can be injected in the first session (two 5-mL vials). The dose should be distributed in the area to be treated and the patient's reaction observed.

From this point on, when treating different body areas at the same time, the physician may inject up to eight vials of 5 mL each during one session. The procedure should be repeated from one to four times, waiting 3 months for the retraction of the skin. Treatment should be continued if necessary. Experience shows that most patients achieve their goals before the last session.

Aging Neck

Lipodissolution is performed in the aging neck as follows:

- Diagnose correctly to inject the subcutaneous area.
- Clean the area along the jaw line and divide it in three points.
- Inject 0.3 mL of Lipostabil in each point.
- If necessary, inject a second parallel line.

- Repeat the procedure every 15 days for at most four sessions.
- Wait 3 months for the retraction of the skin to inject again.
- Advise the patient to wear a compressive strip on the site for the first two nights following treatment.

RESULTS

Lipodissolve does not permanently remove fat cells from the treated area. Some may remain. If the patient gains weight after treatment, the area treated does not tend to increase in size as quickly as it would have if the treatment not been performed. Fat distribution is directed elsewhere as in liposuction. This distribution achieves a better balance in body shape because usually only disproportionate areas are treated. The patient should be instructed not to gain more than 4 kg after the procedure or the results will not last. Because the skin tightens over the treated area as the fat is removed, there is no looseness of skin.

COMPLICATIONS

Clinical experience has shown that not even a single case of complications has been found as long as a qualified physician performs the procedure. Lipodissolution is a safe and effective method of fat reduction when performed by a skilled physician. Unlike liposuction and surgery, it is not associated with the risks of general anesthesia or sedation. No complications or side effects are observed. No downtime is necessary.

REFERENCES

1. Pistor M. Mesotherapie Pratique. Paris: Masson Editeurs; 1998.
2. Warembourg H, Jaillard J. Clinical trial of Lipostabil in the treatment of diabetic angiopatic. Lille Med 1968;13(6):Suppl 727–31.
3. Fiume Z. Final report on the safety assessment of lecithin and hydrogenated lecithin. Int J Toxicol 2001;200(Suppl 1):21–45.
4. Rittes PG. The use of phosphatidylcholine for correction of lower lid bulging due to prominent fat pads. Dermatol Surg 2001;27:391–2.
5. Kirsten R, Heintz B, Nelson K, et al. Reduction of hyperlipidemia with 3-sn-polyenyl-phosphatidylcholine in dialysis patients. Int J Clin Pharmacol Ther Toxicol 1989;27:129–34.
6. Wattel F, Scherpereel P, Sezille G, et al. Use of polyunsaturated phospholipids in the treatment

of fat embolism. Lille Med 1974;19(8 Suppl 3): 870–4.

7. Rittes PG. The use of phosphatidylcholine for correction of localized fat deposits. Aesthetic Plast Surg 2003;27:315–8.

8. Rittes P. The injections of phosphatidylcholine in fat tissue: experimental study of local action in rabbits. Aesthetic Plast Surg 2006;30:474–8.

9. Ablon G, Rotunda AM. Treatment of lower eyelid fat pads using phosphatidylcholine: clinical trial and review. Dermatol Surg 2004;30:422–7.

10. Rotunda AM, Suzuki H, Moy RL, et al. Detergent effects of sodium deoxycholate are a major feature of an injectable phosphatidylcholine formulation used for localized fat dissolution. Dermatol Surg 2004;30:1001–8.

11. Rose PT, Morgan M. Histological changes associated with mesotherapy for fat dissolution. J Cosmet laser Ther 2005;7(1):17–9.

12. Rittes P. Complications of Lipostabil Endovena for treating localized fat deposits. Aesthetic Surg J 2007;27(2):146–9.

Review of "The Lipodissolve Technique: Clinical Experience"

Joseph P. Hunstad, MD, FACS*, Michelle De Souza, MD

KEYWORDS

- Lipodissolve • Injection lipolysis • Mesotherapy
- Phosphatidylcholine • Deoxycholate

Dr. Patricia Rittes is a pioneer of the Lipodissolve technique for injection lipolysis. She has published several articles detailing her experience.[1-3] In this article, we briefly discuss the background of Lipodissolve and the current status of injection lipolysis in the United States, and review Dr. Rittes' results using Lipodissolve on the periorbital fat pads, the neck, and the back.

Injection lipolysis is the generic term for the subcutaneous injection of compounds that break down fat. This technique is referred to as Lipodissolve, Lipostabil, or mesotherapy, among other terms. However, these labels are not truly interchangeable. Lipodissolve, as described by Dr. Rittes, is the nonsurgical technique of fat emulsification by injection of a single compound phosphatidylcholine (PPC). Lipostabil (Sanofi-Aventis, Bridgewater, NJ) is a mixture of PPC and deoxycholate (DC) and has been in use for injection lipolysis for about 12 years. Mesotherapy is the subcutaneous injection of nonspecific compounds to treat a multitude of ailments.

Both compounds, PPC and DC, occur naturally in the body, functioning to break down fat and cholesterol. Although both compounds are used during injection lipolysis, there is some debate regarding which is the active ingredient. In a randomized, double-blinded study by Salti and colleagues[4] comparing injection lipolysis using PPC/DC with using DC alone, DC alone is shown to be equally effective. The prevailing belief is that these agents may work synergistically to improve fat dissolution.

Dr. Rittes uses Lipostabil (Aventis), composed of PPC and DC. This compound is also marketed and studied in Europe, at times under the name, Lipostabil N (Artegodan Pharmacy, Germany).[5] In the United States, PPC/DC is obtained from compounding pharmacies (**Fig. 1**). These pharmacies are not regulated by the US Federal Drug Administration (FDA), but by each individual state.[6] Because of the need to use compounding pharmacies, there is no standard formulation for PPC/DC, allowing for the unregulated addition of vitamins, herbal extracts, and other substances that can cause adverse reactions.[5] The use of PPC/DC for injection lipolysis is considered off-label use.

The FDA has only recently begun reviewing the outcome of patients treated by injection lipolysis. Dr. Leroy Young is conducting the only FDA-approved study of PPC and DC, which is supported by a grant from the Aesthetic Society Education and Research Foundation. Dr. Young is conducting a randomized control trial of 47% PPC and 52% DC versus placebo. Patients are monitored before and after injections by way of photography, sequential measurements of treated areas, MRI, biopsy, Dexa scan, and serum levels. An average treatment dosage is 900 mg, PPC, well below the maximum safe dose of 100 mL of PPC, 2500 mg, PPC.[7] Treatments are repeated at 8 week intervals, allowing for resolution of the inflammatory process. (Leroy Young, MD, personal communication, 2008).

The authors have no disclosures relevant to this manuscript.
The Hunstad Center for Cosmetic Plastic Surgery, P.A., 8605 Cliff Cameron Drive, Suite 100, Charlotte, NC 28269, USA
* Corresponding author.
E-mail address: jph1@hunstadcenter.com (J.P. Hunstad).

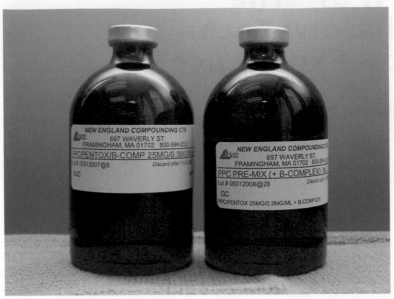

Fig.1. Samples of Lipodissolve obtained from New England Compounding Center. These samples contain different concentrations of PPC/DC, Pentoxifylline, and Vitamin B complex.

Clinically, injection lipolysis carries a significant adverse reaction profile. Immediately after injection, the onset of pain, erythema, edema, pruritis, and warmth belie the intermediate results (**Fig. 2**). Sequelae of the injection last from 15 minutes to 72 hours,[1] with localized injection site sensitivity that can last for 1 month.[7] The process may be repeated as frequently as every other week with an encore of the same side effects. Although a marginal improvement may occur after one treatment, we have observed that the initial pain, swelling, and bruising often inhibits patients from enduring the further treatments necessary

for an optimal result. For those patients who do return for more injections, the inflammatory process is equally profound, again calling into question the arduous journey to reach the desired endpoint.

Dr. Young relates that patients display immediate mild swelling and bruising with modest pain. Anecdotally, Dr. Young has noticed that treating thicker tissue such as the periumbilical region is less painful, whereas thinner tissue near the anterior superior iliac spine results in more pain (Leroy Young, MD, personal communication, 2008). Our experience echoes that of Dr. Young.

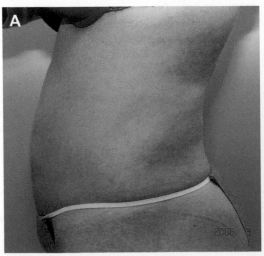
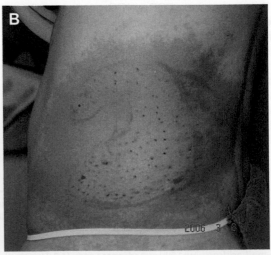

Fig. 2. A patient's left flank before (A) and 45 minutes after (B) application of Lipodissolve. Expansive erythema and edema are immediately apparent.

Dr. Rittes shows significant improvement in the periorbital fat pads in three patients after two, four, and six treatments of Lipodissolve, respectively. Although she reports no complications with this procedure, there are concerns of ocular complications such as retro-orbital bleeding.[8] Duncan and Palmer[6] called injections to the lower eyelid fat pad ineffective and fraught with risk. In

the interest of safety, Network Lipolysis, a European scientific organization, has eliminated the lower lid fat pad from the list of lipolysis indications, further adding that only physicians who are capable of treating a retro-orbital hemorrhage should perform injection lipolysis to this area.[8]

Our results have been less successful in treating the periorbital fat pads. One patient who underwent

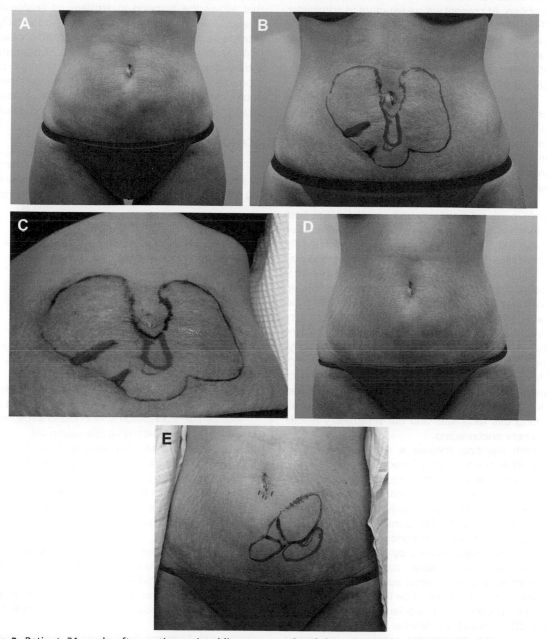

Fig. 3. Patient, 21 weeks after suction-assisted lipectomy to the abdomen. (*A*) She elected touch-up Lipodissolve to the abdomen. (*B*) Pretreatment markings. (*C*) The reaction to Lipodissolve 45 minutes after treatment. (*D*) The patient returned for her second treatment 18 weeks after the first application of Lipodissolve. (*E*) The residual areas to be treated.

injection of PPC/DC into periorbital fat pads noted immediate intense periorbital edema. This edema persisted for months, making her results unsatisfactory. This patient required correction with a lower blepharoplasty 10 months later.

The results shown by Dr. Rittes deserve commendation; although, of note, one of her results has been published in a number of other manuscripts.[1,9] Perhaps this attests to the fact that remarkable results are unusual and difficult to obtain. At present we are reluctant to administer PPC/DC to the periorbita, opting for standard surgical treatment to include transconjunctival blepharoplasty with treatment of fat pads and either skin pinch blepharoplasty, or laser or chemical resurfacing to the skin.

The remaining results shown by Dr. Rittes are less dramatic. One patient underwent 20 sessions to treat localized fat on the back from chronic cortisone therapy. After predictable morbidity and discomfort with each injection, treating a larger area requires a strong commitment from both the patient and treating physician (**Fig. 3**).

In the article by Dr. Rittes, the two patients who had Lipodissolve therapy to the neck have at best a modest improvement in their neck contour. For these patients, treating only the fat did not fully correct the deformity. Ideally, the skin, fat, and platysma should be addressed to achieve an optimal result; a shortfall of the Lipodissolve technique. We have not employed PPC/DC in treating the neck, relying on proven and consistent results using suction-assisted lipectomy, corset platysmaplasty, and skin lifting procedures. Recently, the Smart Lipo MPX laser (Cynosure, Westford, MA) has become available and preliminary results suggest considerable contour improvement and skin tightening of the neck. We are currently evaluating this technique and our preliminary results are very encouraging.

With injection lipolysis a relatively new field, societies have been formed for the scientific advancement of this technique. These organizations, such as Network Lipolysis and American Society for Aesthetic Lipodissolve recommend that only trained physicians perform lipolysis therapy.[8] Workshops designed to teach this technique exist, administered by experienced physicians with reasonable hands-on training.[10] Devastating complications such as skin necrosis have occurred with injection lipolysis by inexperienced persons.[5,6] Physicians who administer PPC/DC should be familiar with, and able to perform, the treatments necessary to correct potential complications. Furthermore, as the long-term effect of Lipodissolve is not known, physicians and patients should proceed with caution. Appropriate informed consent is highly recommended for using this controversial therapy.

Clinically, the idea of treating localized fat deposits in a nonsurgical fashion is appealing to many surgeons and patients who wish to avoid the downtime and perceived risks involved with invasive surgical procedures. Although many physicians have demonstrated success using Lipodissolve, currently we favor the results provided by a properly performed, single-stage surgery that allows the surgeon to address all anatomic levels. Furthermore, surgery can potentially provide a single exposure to morbidity and consistent results, as opposed to multiple treatments with variable results and several exposures to morbidity. Further study and randomized controlled trials are ongoing and necessary before widespread use of Lipodissolve can be endorsed.

ACKNOWLEDGMENTS

The authors would like to thank Dr. Leroy Young for his contribution to this article; and Meena Patel, RN for her assistance with Lipodissolve injections.

REFERENCES

1. Rittes PG. The use of phosphatidylcholine for correction of lower lid bulging due to prominent fat pads. Dermatol Surg 2001;27(4):391–2.
2. Rittes PG. The use of phosphatidylcholine for correction of localized fat deposits. Aesthetic Plast Surg 2003;27(4):315–8.
3. Rittes PG, Rittes JC, Carriel Amary MF, et al. Injection of phosphatidylcholine in fat tissue: experimental study of local action in rabbits. Aesthetic Plast Surg 2006;30(4):474–8.
4. Salti G, Ghersetich I, Tantussi F, et al. Phosphatidylcholine and sodium deoxycholate in the treatment of localized fat: a double-blind, randomized study. Dermatol Surg 2008;34(1):60–6 [discussion 66].
5. Mann MW, Palm MD, Sengelmann RD, et al. New advances in liposuction technology. Semin Cutan Med Surg 2008;27(1):72–82.
6. Duncan DI, Palmer M. Fat reduction using phosphatidylcholine/sodium deoxycholate injections: standard of practice. Aesthetic Plast Surg 2008;32(6):858–72.
7. Duncan DI, Hasengschwandtner F. Lipodissolve for subcutaneous fat reduction and skin retraction. Aesthet Surg J 2005;25:530–43.
8. Hasengschwandtner F. Phosphatidylcholine treatment to induce lipolysis. J Cosmet Dermatol 2005; 4(4):308–13.
9. Young VL. Lipostabil: the effect of phosphatidylcholine on subcutaneous fat. Aesthet Surg J 2003;23:413–7.
10. Available at: www.network-lipolysis.com. Accessed August 2008.

Author's Comment

Patrícia Guedes Rittes, MD

In response to Dr. Hunstad's comments about my article on Lipodissolve, I would like to make the following observations.

The Lipodissolve technique was developed for people who do not want to undergo surgery but would very like much to improve their tired-looking eyes. The technique is not indicated for obese people. Dr. Hunstad refers to publications about a patient who had more than 20 sessions. That patient had Cushing syndrome and was not able to lose even 1 pound with other treatments.

Retrobulbar bleeding has been exhaustively discussed in the literature. When you inject with a needle, it is impossible to cut the vein. This is unlike the situation with blepharoplasty, where it is possible to have bleeding after surgery. In my experience with the Lipodissolve technique, the needle can touch the vein and hurt it, but never cuts the vein.

I have never seen a published paper about necrosis after injections, although I have heard about this occurrence.

I have approximately 13 years' experience of long-term effects.

Santa Casa de Misericórdia Medical School, São Paulo, Brazil
E-mail address: prittes@terra.com.br

Clin Plastic Surg 36 (2009) 227
doi:10.1016/j.cps.2008.12.005
0094-1298/08/$ – see front matter © 2009 Published by Elsevier Inc.

Surgisis Acellular Collagen Matrix in Aesthetic and Reconstructive Plastic Surgery Soft Tissue Applications

Robert F. Centeno, MD, MBA

KEYWORDS

- Surgisis • Acellular collagen matrix • Plastic surgery
- Tissue engineering • Aesthetic surgery
- Surgisis facial implant (SFI)

Surgisis acellular collagen matrix was made commercially available in 1998 soon after Food and Drug Administration (FDA) 510 K clearance for soft tissue reconstruction. Since then, numerous applications have received FDA 510 K clearance of the engineered device. Application of this porcine intestinal mucosa–derived device in plastic surgery applications has been recent. Several IRB–approved studies are currently in progress to assess the long-term performance in aesthetic and reconstructive breast surgery and aesthetic facial rejuvenation. To date, some limited longer-term data are becoming available that support the use of Surgisis in plastic surgery applications.

BASIC SCIENCE AND BACKGROUND

Surgisis is manufactured from a readily available, abundant extracellular matrix (ECM) material derived from the submucosal layer of the pig small intestine, also referred to as small intestinal submucosa, or SIS.[1] The submucosa is the layer of connective tissue that provides strength to the pig small intestine. It is approximately 100 to 200 μm thick, and in the living intestine it supports the growth and differentiation of the mucosal and glandular cells while maintaining a connective tissue structure that gives the intestine its integrity.

Like dermis or fascia, the small intestinal submucosa is composed of fibrillar collagens and adhesive glycoproteins, which serve as a scaffold into which cells can migrate and multiply. Because of its importance in the constant renewal of the multitude of cell types in the intestine, the ECM of the small intestine also contains potent regulatory factors, such as glycosaminoglycans, proteoglycans, and growth factors. These factors help regulate cellular processes that maintain tissue homeostasis and respond to injury and infection.

Unlike allografts or autografts, which are not subject to stringent regulatory oversight to ensure safety, xenograft materials must be purified to ensure safety. Surgisis is manufactured by mechanically separating the submucosa from its outer muscular layers and internal mucosal layers, treating it to remove cells and cellular debris, and subjecting it to robust disinfection methods to eliminate the risk for disease transmission.[2] Unlike acellular cadaveric dermis, it is then terminally sterilized using ethylene oxide gas. When implanted surgically, it stimulates angiogenesis, connective and epithelial tissue growth and

Dr. Centeno participates in the Speaker's Bureau and performs contracted research for Cook Biotech, Inc., the manufacturer of Surgisis.
St. Croix Plastic Surgery and MediSpa, St. Croix, VI, USA
E-mail address: rfcenteno@gmail.com

doi:10.1016/j.cps.2008.12.004

differentiation, and deposition, organization, and maturation of ECM components that are functionally and histologically appropriate to the site of implantation.[1,3,4]

Surgisis is unique among biologic graft materials because the signaling components that make the ECM an interactive structure are retained through the entire manufacturing process. For example, it has been shown to contain potent regulatory factors, such as glycosaminoglycans, proteoglycans, and growth factors, which regulate cellular processes that maintain tissue homeostasis and respond to injury.[5] It has been shown to recruit marrow-derived stem cells to the area of implant,[6] protect bioactive factors from a proteolytic wound environment,[7] and stimulate cultured cells to secrete their own growth factors, which further aids in tissue restoration.[7,8] In animal models of angiogenesis, Surgisis has been proven to rapidly stimulate blood vessel growth to allow it early access to the patient's immune system, providing a possible mechanism by which Surgisis can withstand implantation in contaminated fields.[9]

Surgisis has been used in various surgical applications. In animals, SIS was first used in the vascular system to experimentally replace superior vena cava and aorta.[10,11] Since that time, it has been shown to be effective in restoring functional innervation and smooth muscle cell contractility in the injured canine bladder.[12] It has also been examined in long-term canine studies of experimental body wall replacement. In these studies, it was demonstrated to maintain its strength out to an endpoint of 2 years[13] and to result in lesser degrees of chronic inflammation and greater amounts of collagen and muscle cell differentiation than other graft materials.[14]

In humans, products based on the submucosa technology have been used to treat more than 500,000 patients in fields ranging from wound care to colorectal surgery, to hernia and pelvic floor repair, and even to plastic and cosmetic surgery. In randomized clinical wound care trials, the OASIS Wound Matrix was shown to be superior to conventional compression therapy alone in leading to complete healing of venous stasis ulcers within 12 weeks.[15] It was also shown to be equally as effective as expensive growth factor treatment in leading to complete closure of diabetic foot ulcers.[16] In a European randomized clinical trial against Hyaloskin (a purified hyaluronic acid product), treatment of mixed arteriovenous ulcers with OASIS led to complete closure in 83% of ulcers as compared with 46% of those treated with Hyaloskin. Taken together, these studies indicate that products based on the SIS technology can be effective in healing chronic skin wounds, and suggest that the complex composition of all products based on this technology plays a role in their efficacy.

In no single application does the composition of Surgisis and its ability to quickly interact with patient tissues play a more critical role than when it is placed in potentially contaminated or contaminated fields. Even though success varies based on the degree of infection and the type of microorganism present, in many of these cases traditional synthetic meshes cannot be ethically used because it has been well established that they become infected and need to later be removed: two well-documented uses include anal fistula repair and complex hernia repair.

In anorectal fistulas, the Surgisis material has been documented repeatedly to result in effective fistula closure within approximately 3 months of placement (see Refs.[17-19]). Multiple published case series report healing rates at 3 months in excess of 70%,[17-23] whereas others report only a 24% to 46% healing rate.[23-27] The major difference between these series was that the lower success rates seemed to be related to the presence of overt abscesses in the fistula tracts and the application of Surgisis in tracts that had repeatedly failed other procedures. The Surgisis material fared better in cases of contamination as compared with cases of overt infection, and in cases that were more acute as compared with more chronic fistulas that had failed multiple other procedures. It is obvious that in the cases in which Surgisis fails, no other graft materials are likely to succeed either.

Surgisis has an extensive history of use in various hernia repair procedures. In inguinal hernia repair, it has been shown to be effective and durable to more than 3 years when used with tacks or fibrin glue.[28] It has been effective in returning athletes to the field quickly in cases of "sports hernia," wherein groin pain is experienced but a hernia is not confirmed.[29] It has also been shown to result in less chronic pain than synthetics in this location, and has been effective even in immunocompromised patients.[30] In a prospective, randomized trial of large paraesophageal hernias, it significantly reduced the rate of early recurrence when used as a bolster,[31] and in ventral hernia repair it has effectively resulted in long-term retention of domain for as long as 5 years.[9]

The most challenging locations in which to use Surgisis are grossly contaminated hernias, where any surgical repair is likely to result in complications. When using Surgisis in grossly contaminated cases, Helton and colleagues[32] suggest a staged repair strategy and caution its use in dirty wounds or in critically ill patients if a staged strategy is not used. They suggest that the avoidance of closed-space infection adjacent to the Surgisis material is important for long-term efficacy and that prevention of colonization at the time of implantation should prevent delayed infections from occurring. They further note that their best results were achieved when they were able to minimize seroma or hematoma formation and prevent infection between the mesh and the peritoneal cavity. It is likely that maintaining contact of the mesh with vascularized tissue is essential to a satisfactory outcome. In their experience, fewer complications were noted with laparoscopic placement of the Surgisis than with open placement, but when open repair was needed in the presence of contamination, they suggested the use of Surgisis as an inlay prosthesis without completely closing the wound, making liberal use of wet-to-dry dressings and vacuum-assisted closure until the contamination was resolved, and then subsequently placing a skin graft if necessary to achieve complete closure.

PLASTIC SURGERY APPLICATIONS
Breast Reconstruction

The use of biologic implants in reconstructive breast surgery is a recent innovation in plastic surgery. Breunig and Warren[33] initially reported the use of human cadaveric allografts in reconstructing the inframammary crease and to allow immediate single-stage breast reconstruction with an alloplastic implant in 2005. Subsequently, multiple authors have reported its use in the same application in immediate breast reconstruction with tissue expanders. This technique allows for a more natural and efficient expander/implant reconstruction than either the complete submuscular or partial submuscular reconstruction technique. The complication rates of this new technique also seem to be comparable to published series of tissue expander breast reconstruction. Its success and popularity have led to rapid adoption of this relatively new technique.

The cost-prohibitive nature of using multiple pieces of cadaveric human dermis remains a significant concern and reason for pause. Additionally, the inconvenience of having to suture pieces of cadaveric human or porcine dermis together to achieve complete expander coverage led the author to seek an engineered biologic implant alternative. Surgisis EXL biologic mesh is an FDA-approved product with indications for soft tissue reconstruction, the indication for which it was intended in this application. This engineered product is cost effective in nature, readily available in large sizes, and easy to use.

After complete informed consent was obtained, patients who were deemed candidates for immediate tissue expander reconstruction were reconstructed using a Surgisis EXL 5 × 30 cm biologic mesh suture to the previously marked inframammary crease position and to the inferior border of the detached pectoralis. Complete coverage of the expander was achieved in all cases (**Fig. 1**). The procedure was performed similarly to the previously published technique. The patient in **Fig. 2** demonstrates the efficacy and applicability of Surgisis biologic implants in this soft tissue reconstruction application. **Table 1** documents the outcomes associated with its use in different applications.

Mastopexy—Internal Suspension

The use of internal suspension sutures and mesh in mastopexy surgery has been well documented in the literature. The recurrence of skin laxity leading to parenchymal descent in the long term is a vexing problem experienced by many plastic surgeons in the United States. Outside the United States, the use of alloplastic permanent and absorbable mesh has been popularized by Sampaio-Goes.[34,35] His long-term results support the efficacy of internal mesh suspension in prolonging the results of the mastopexy procedure. Concerns about the impact of alloplastic mesh in confounding the results of screening mammography and the potential for litigation has delayed the widespread adoption of its use in this application. Mastopexy is another application for soft tissue reconstruction in which an engineered, cost-effective biologic

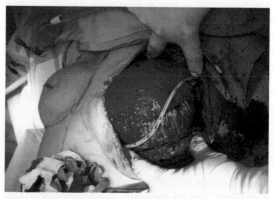

Fig. 1. Intraoperative view of Surgisis EXL 5 × 30 cm graft in an immediate tissue expander reconstruction. The graft is sutured in place to the inframammary fold; the lateral axillary fascia and the inferior border of the detached pectoralis major providing complete implant coverage.

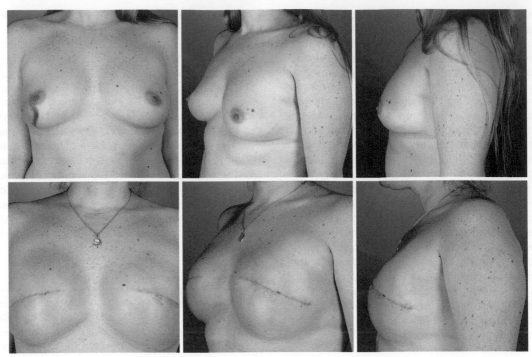

Fig. 2. A 45–year-old patient shown 8 months after bilateral mastectomy and immediate breast reconstruction with Surgisis EXL 5 × 30 cm graft and a tissue expander followed by replacement with a permanent implant and nipple areola reconstruction.

implant like Surgisis seems to have a role. Its incorporation and replacement by the host's tissue should allay the concerns about mammographic alteration. The author is unaware of any evidence in the literature that cadaveric or xenogenic biologic implants have oncogenic potential. The cadaveric and porcine dermal products, while similarly effective, have the disadvantage of being cost prohibitive in cosmetic applications and cumbersome to use because of size limitations. Although the author's long-term results in this application are limited, the device seems to have usefulness in this application (**Figs 3** and **4**). Its efficacy in prolonging the therapeutic effect of a mastopexy is deserving of further study in a systematic and objective way. Controlled studies in bilateral procedures are difficult to perform from a practical and an ethical standpoint.

Nasolabial, Labiomandibular, Glabellar Folds

The treatment of nasolabial, labiomandibular, and glabellar folds has long been managed with injectable fillers. The off-the-shelf convenience and relative safety of these devices have made them popular with consumers. Unfortunately, the significant volume of fillers required to achieve a good clinical result and the longevity of the fillers remain economic concerns for most patients. "Filler

fatigue" among patients is not an uncommon finding in many aesthetic practices. Although the noninvasive and low-downtime nature of these treatments make them popular early on, the average patient frequently tires of the cost of repeated treatments. This fatigue has led companies to develop fillers of longer duration and even some that purport to be permanent. Although the author feels that the quest for a permanent filler is likely misguided, longer-lasting fillers that are cost effective for patients would certainly be welcome in the market. Surgisis acellular collagen matrix grafts seem to potentially fit this niche. Although a surgical procedure is required to treat these areas, Surgisis strands or cylinders can be deployed in various subcutaneous planes to get good soft tissue augmentation and correction (**Fig. 5**). The longevity of these treatments still requires thorough documentation, but early results in a small series of patients are promising (**Figs. 6–9**). Its cost effectiveness also makes it competitive with fillers and more cost effective than cadaveric or other xenogenic grafts. Formal study of the longevity of the device in the treatment of nasolabial folds is currently in progress.

Neck Suspension Sling

The use of sutures and devices to perform a minimally invasive neck lift or as an adjunct to open

Table 1
Results

Location	Breast	Nasolabial Folds	Labiomandibular Folds	Glabellar Folds	Premaxillary, Premandibular	Neck	Abdomen
No. of patients	5	17	2	2	1	1	1
No. of devices	9	146	4	4	3	1	1
No. of seromas	1	—	—	—	—	—	—
No. of infections	—	2	—	1	—	—	1
No. of removals	—	1	—	1	—	1	—
Visibility	—	—	—	—	—	1	—
Palpability	—	16	2	2	3	1	1

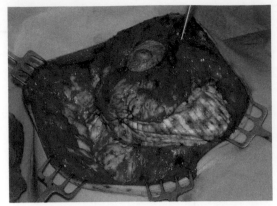

Fig. 3. Intraoperative view of internal suspension of breast parenchyma in a vertical short scar mastopexy.

neck and face lift procedure is a fertile area of investigation and marketing today. Various devices have been used in this application, including Surgisis. The drawback of the current techniques available is the edema and ridge effect that persists after these procedures (**Figs. 10** and **11**). Although this problem is likely self-limited and is possibly technique related, in the author's experience all of the devices used in this application seem to suffer from the same drawback. Neck procedures have a significant amount of dependent edema independent of the use of fixation devices. This application is one in which surgical intervention still seems to

provide the best solution with the fastest recovery and fewest complications.

Lip Augmentation

Pribitkin and colleagues[36] reported the use of Surgisis acellular collagen matrix in lip augmentation. Eight patients underwent augmentation with 1×6 cm strips and were followed for 6 months. Four of the eight patients were satisfied with the outcome and four patients desired further augmentation. Adverse events included transient erythema and cellulitis in one patient that resolved with oral antibiotics. The author has no personal clinical experience with the device in this application. Given the average aesthetic patient's desire for a short recovery, this procedure seems applicable in lip augmentation patients who have filler fatigue and tolerance for potential morbidity. Our inability as surgeons to achieve effective long-lasting lip augmentation with existing techniques supports further study of this procedure.

Premaxillary Augmentation

Augmentation of the premaxilla has been performed with calcium hydroxyapatite, bone grafts, soft tissue grafts, and alloplastic implants. Today, it is most commonly performed in cosmetic rhinoplasty surgery wherein the patient presents with a hidden columella due to premaxillary bony and

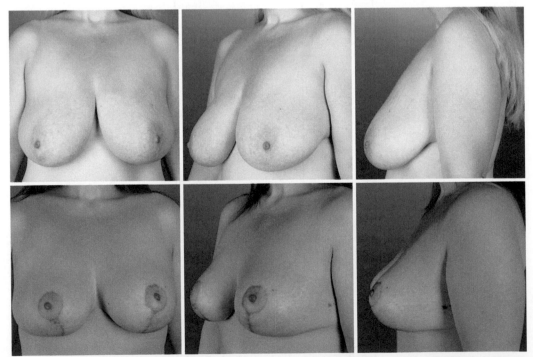

Fig. 4. A 35-year-old patient shown 4 months after vertical short scar mastopexy with Surgisis EXL 5×30 cm graft internal parenchymal suspension.

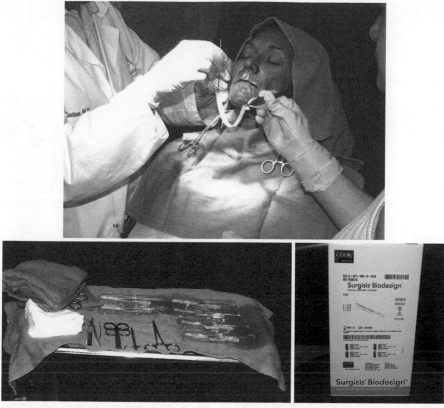

Fig. 5. Nasolabial fold correction with Surgisis 1 × 6 cm facial strips under local anesthesia.

soft tissue deficiency. This procedure is often done by constructing either an autogenous or an allo-pathic graft to fit the application. The availability of a cost-effective, engineered implant certainly is an efficient way of addressing this need. The longevity of the soft tissue correction in this application is unknown, but its efficacy is supported by the results shown in **Fig. 12**.

Nipple Reconstruction

Although long-term data are not yet available, nipple reconstruction in post-oncologic breast reconstruction is an application in which Surgisis cylinders may be applicable. Although a plethora of techniques have been described to produce natural, long-term results there is no consensus regarding the best approach to this vexing recon-structive problem. Early results are favorable with virtually all reconstructive techniques, but the long-term results fail to show persistence in most cases. Attempts at addressing this problem with acellular human dermis and injectable fillers show good short-term success, but marginal long-term results. The unanswered question is whether using an acellular collagen biologically active matrix cylinder to stent the reconstructive

flaps will provide for long-term persistence of nipple projection. Off-the-shelf Surgisis nipple reconstruction cylinders are available that show anecdotally good results, but long-term reports are still pending.

TECHNICAL CONSIDERATIONS

As with any implant, there are many factors that affect the success of its placement. Host factors, such as whether the surgical site is infected or contaminated, the site has been irradiated, or the patient is undergoing chemotherapy, all are relevant to the success of the procedure. Whether an implant is alloplastic, xenogenic, homologous, or autologous, all of these factors can deleteriously affect the outcome. The use of Surgisis SIS acel-lular collagen matrix is no exception to these basic tenets. Although Surgisis SIS does show some resistance to infection, optimally the implant should be placed in a noninfected or contaminated site. This placement is especially relevant in aesthetic applications in the face. Placement of a facial implant in patients who have active acne, pustules, or fever blisters should be avoided until these conditions are under control. Although the

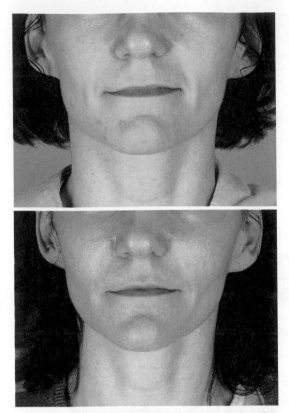

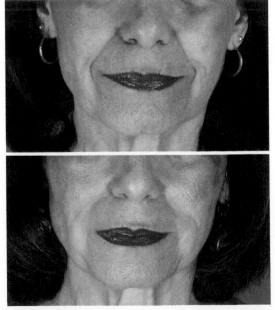

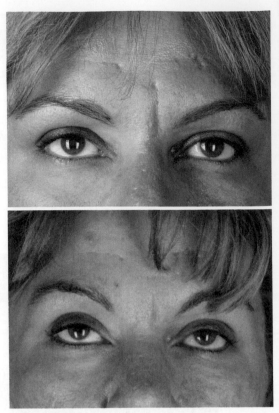

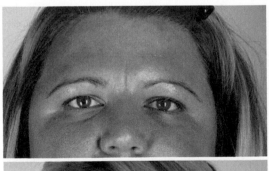

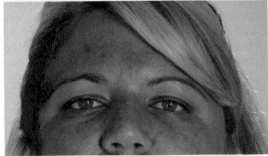

Fig. 6. A 38-year-old patient shown 8 months after nasolabial fold correction with Surgisis 1 × 6 cm facial strips under local anesthesia.

Fig. 7. A 69-year-old patient shown 11 months after nasolabial fold correction with Surgisis 2 × 15 cm facial strips under local anesthesia.

Fig. 8. A 40-year-old patient shown 12 months after glabellar fold correction with Surgisis 1 × 6 cm facial strips under local anesthesia and adjunctive treatment with Botox.

Fig. 9. A 31-year-old patient shown 12 months after glabellar fold correction with Surgisis 1 × 6 cm facial strips under local anesthesia and adjunctive treatment with Botox.

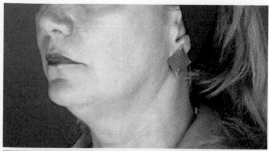

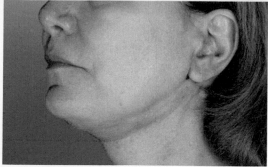

Fig. 10. A 54-year-old patient shown 1 month after neck lift with internal neck suspension with 2 × 30 cm Surgisis strip anchored to the mastoid fascia. Note the erythema, edema, and banding around the suspension sling.

author has successfully placed the implant in a remotely radiated breast, placement in tissue with recent or planned future radiation should be avoided. Planned chemotherapy is not an absolute contraindication for use, but its impact on healing, infection, and implant complications should be considered.

Handling of the Surgisis SIS acellular collagen matrix implant is important to optimal outcomes. As with the placement of any implant, minimizing

handling of the implant and contact with the skin is important in avoiding contamination and colonization with skin flora. Hydration of the implant for the appropriate length of time (neither over- nor underhydration) is also important to timely incorporation. Surgisis can be hydrated in saline containing antibiotics. The manufacturer recommends hydration in cefazolin and bacitracin, but vancomycin, clindamycin, and gentamicin should be avoided. Additionally, using latex-free gloves during placement is recommended by the manufacturer. The implant should be handled with sterile instruments as much as possible.

When placing the implants in the face, care should be taken to place the implant in the subcutaneous tissue and not immediately subdermal to avoid visibility. The ends of the implant should either be trimmed or meticulously buried in a subcutaneous pocket to avoid extrusion of the implant. Another technical matter is placement of the entrance and exit incisions. To treat the nasolabial fold, one incision should be in the nasolabial fold and one incision should be at the border of the mandible in the prejowl area. If the incision is placed at the end of the nasolabial fold, the incision will be visible for a prolonged period of time because of postinflammatory hyperpigmentation and dependent edema. In treating the labiomandibular fold, the oral commissure and the mandibular border should be used as incision locations. In the glabella, the incisions are placed at the end of the fold and the implant ends are buried in a small 0.5-cm pocket that extends beyond the ends of the incisions. Unfortunately, visibility of the incision is unavoidable in the glabella area and patients should be counseled that they will have to conceal it with make-up until it fades. Adjunctive Botox before treatment and limited subcision under

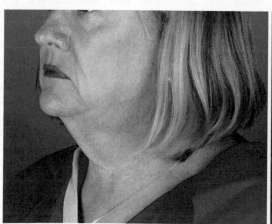

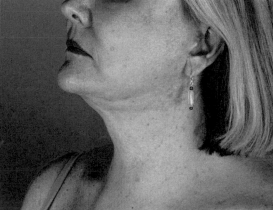

Fig. 11. A 52-year-old patient shown 1 month after neck lift with internal neck suspension with Endotine Ribbon anchored to the mastoid fascia. Note the erythema, edema, and banding around the suspension sling.

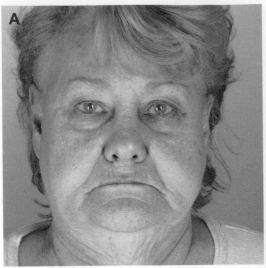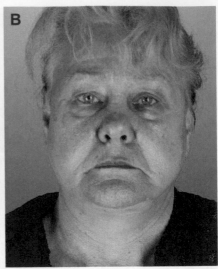

Fig. 12. A 66-year-old patient shown before (A) and 10.5 months after (B) face lift with platysmal placation, facial resurfacing, nasolabial, labiomandibular fold correction with Surgisis 1 × 6 cm facial strips and Surgisis 0.4 × 10 cm facial cylinders and premaxillary/premandibular augmentation with Surgisis 0.4 × 10 cm facial cylinder.

glabellar folds also enhances the outcome in this area. Fortunately, with Surgisis SFI implants there is no risk for embolization associated with injectable fillers or autologous fat in this anatomic area.

Use of Surgisis SIS mesh either in the breast or abdomen requires several strategies to minimize the risk for seroma formation. Reducing dead space in the surgical field with compression and closed suction drainage are important strategies. In the breast, drains are used when Surgisis is applied as in internal sling during mastopexy. In breast reconstruction with expanders and inferior Surgisis sling, the expander is typically filled to approximately 50% of the projected final fill volume based on the weight of the mastectomy specimen. Any redundant skin-sparing mastectomy skin is resected in patients who have pendulous breasts. One to two hubless Blake drains are place to further reduce dead space. Finally, gentle external compression with a fluff dressing and support bra is applied. The drains are left in place until the output is less than 30 mL in 24 hours. Expansion of the expander before drain removal is also helpful in reducing dead space and avoiding seromas. Given the high complication rates associated with tissue expander reconstructions, there is no substitute for sound clinical judgment in this application. In the abdomen, use of closed suction drainage and external compression also helps to reduce the risk for a seroma.

OUTCOMES

Surgisis SIS has many potential applications in plastic and reconstructive surgery. To date, this series of 29 patients is the largest series on the use of Surgisis SIS published in the plastic surgery literature (**Table 1**). This series documents the success of the device in facial rejuvenation surgery, reconstructive and aesthetic breast surgery, and body contouring surgery.

Of the 29 patients, all but 2 are very satisfied with the treatments. The 2 patients who were not completely satisfied were 1 neck lift patient who had prolonged erythema, induration, and visibility of the implant, and 1 nasolabial fold augmentation patient who had a unilateral infection. Both patients had the implants removed without further incident and with complete resolution of their problems.

There were a total of four presumptive infections in the series. One patient had a culture-positive wound infection after abdominoplasty with hernia repair and abdominal wall reinforcement with a 35 × 35 cm Surgisis EXL implant. This patient responded well to oral antibiotics and the implant was left in place. She recovered uneventfully. One glabella fold patient had a culture-positive infection and was treated with oral antibiotics and had the implant removed. One nasolabial fold patient had unilateral erythema that responded to oral antibiotics. She recovered uneventfully and the implant was left in place. The infection rate is thus 4/29 patients (13%) or 4/168 devices or (2%). This finding may reflect the small number of patients in the series. The implants were only removed for infection in two of the four cases, supporting the contention that the biomaterial is resistant to infection. All four patients ultimately had good cosmetic outcomes despite the complications.

Seromas have been reported to be a concern with the use of Surgisis SIS in the general surgery literature. This concern seems to be relevant in plastic surgery procedures in which the implant is placed in a surgical field with dead space. Use of the biomaterial in these cases makes the use of closed suction drainage imperative. Furthermore, compression after drain removal is also helpful in mitigating this problem. In abdominal and breast cases, closed suction drainage and external compression make this issue manageable, but it remains a concern. The use of the Surgisis SIS strip as reinforcement and suspension in a neck lift either through a minimally invasive approach or by way of an open procedure has been problematic in the author's hands. The paucity of tissue to conceal the implant, the dependency of the surgical field, and the dead space present technical challenges for application of this novel biomaterial. The advantages of using an internal suspension sling seem to be outweighed by the increased morbidity in this application.

The area that seems to hold great promise for the application of Surgisis is in facial soft tissue augmentation, namely glabella, labiomandibular, and nasolabial folds. Soft tissue augmentation to the premaxilla is also promising. The devices can be deployed in multiple subcutaneous planes with good success and soft tissue augmentation. The lack of dead space makes seromas virtually nonexistent. The persistence of the soft tissue correction is also promising. Patients continue to show persistence of the correction up to 1 year later. Prospective trials are currently underway to measure this persistence in a more standardized fashion. The implants are rarely visible if deployed meticulously, but prolonged palpability is an issue. Before incorporation occurs, the implant can be palpated through the skin. If patients are adequately counseled regarding this issue, they rarely find it objectionable. They are uniformly satisfied with the outcome if expectations are appropriately managed.

SUMMARY

Tissue engineering in aesthetic and reconstructive plastic surgery remains an elusive goal. The advent of Surgisis extracellular collagen matrix and its performance characteristics suggest that the use of a bioengineered tissue substitute can meet some of our reconstructive requirements. Incorporation and replacement by host tissue with minimal allergic or immune response seems to be achievable today. The ability to engineer the device, the ready availability of substrate, and its cost effectiveness support the use of Surgisis in aesthetic and reconstructive plastic surgery applications. Future product innovations and engineering seem promising. The permanent role of Surgisis in aesthetic and reconstructive plastic surgery will be determined by its documented long-term performance.

REFERENCES

1. Badylak SF. Small intestinal submucosa (SIS): a biomaterial conducive to smart tissue remodeling. In: Bell E, editor. Tissue engineering: current perspectives. Cambridge (MA): Burkhauser; 1993. p. 179–89.
2. Hodde JP, Hiles MC. Virus safety of a porcine-derived medical device: evaluation of a viral inactivation method. Biotechnol Bioeng 2002;79:211–6.
3. Sandusky GE, Badylak SF, Morff RJ, et al. Histologic findings after in vivo placement of small intestinal submucosal vascular grafts and saphenous vein grafts in the carotid artery in dogs. Am J Pathol 1992;140:317–24.
4. Kropp BP, Rippy MK, Badylak SF, et al. Regenerative urinary bladder augmentation using small intestinal submucosa: urodynamic and histopathologic assessment in long term canine bladder augmentations. J Urol 1996;155:2098–104.
5. Hodde J, Janis A, Ernst D, et al. Effects of sterilization on an extracellular matrix scaffold: part I. Composition and matrix architecture. J Mater Sci Mater Med 2007;18:537–43.
6. Badylak SF, Park K, Peppas N, et al. Marrow-derived cells populate scaffolds composed of xenogeneic extracellular matrix. Exp Hematol 2001;29:1310–8.
7. Nihsen ES, Zopf DA, Ernst DMJ, et al. Absorption of bioactive molecules into OASIS wound matrix. Adv Skin Wound Care 2007;20:541–8.
8. Hodde JP, Allam R. Extracellular wound matrices: small intestinal submucosa wound matrix for chronic wound healing. Wounds 2007;19:157–62.
9. Franklin ME Jr, Treviño JM, Portillo G, et al. The use of porcine small intestinal submucosa as a prosthetic material for laparoscopic hernia repair in infected and potentially contaminated fields: long-term follow-up. Surg Endosc 2008;22:1941–6.
10. Lantz GC, Badylak SF, Coffey AC, et al. Small intestinal submucosa as a superior vena cava graft in the dog. J Surg Res 1992;53:175–81.
11. Badylak SF, Lantz GC, Coffey A, et al. Small intestinal submucosa as a large diameter vascular graft in the dog. J Surg Res 1989;47:74–80.
12. Kropp BP. Developmental aspects of the contractile smooth muscle component in small intestinal submucosa regenerated urinary bladder. In: Baskin, Hayward, editors. Advances in bladder research.

New York: Kluwer Academic/Plenum Publishers; 1999. p. 129–35.

13. Badylak SF, Kokini K, Tullius B, et al. Strength over time of a resorbable bioscaffold for body wall repair in a dog model. J Surg Res 2001;99:282–7.

14. Badylak S, Kokini K, Tullius B, et al. Morphologic study of small intestinal submucosa as a body wall repair device. J Surg Res 2002;103:190–202.

15. Mostow EN, Haraway GD, Dalsing M, et al. Effectiveness of an extracellular matrix graft (OASIS Wound Matrix) in the treatment of chronic leg ulcers: a randomized clinical trial. J Vasc Surg 2005;41: 837–43.

16. Niezgoda JA, Van Gils CC, Frykberg RG, et al. Randomized clinical trial comparing OASIS Wound Matrix to Regranex Gel for diabetic ulcers. Adv Skin Wound Care 2005;18:258–66.

17. Johnson EK, Gaw JU, Armstrong DN. Efficacy of anal fistula plug vs. fibrin glue in closure of anorectal fistulas. Dis Colon Rectum 2006;49:371–6.

18. O'Connor L, Champagne BJ, Ferguson MA, et al. Efficacy of anal fistula plug in closure of Crohn's anorectal fistulas. Dis Colon Rectum 2006;49:1569–73.

19. Champagne BJ, O'Connor LM, Ferguson M, et al. Efficacy of anal fistula plug in closure of cryptoglandular fistulas: long-term follow-up. Dis Colon Rectum 2006;49:1817–21.

20. Ellis CN. Bioprosthetic plugs for complex anal fistulas: an early experience. J Surg Educ 2007;64:36–40.

21. Ky AJ, Sylla P, Steinhagen E, et al. Collagen fistula plug for the treatment of anal fistulas. Dis Colon Rectum 2008;51:838–43.

22. Garg P. To determine the efficacy of anal fistula plug in the treatment of high fistula-in-ano—an initial experience. Colorectal Dis 2008 Jul 15; [Epub].

23. Schwandner O, Stadler F, Dietl O, et al. Initial experience on efficacy in closure of cryptoglandular and Crohn's transsphincteric fistulas by the use of the anal fistula plug. Int J Colorectal Dis 2008;23:319–24.

24. van Koperen PJ, D'Hoore A, Wolthuis AM, et al. Anal fistula plug for closure of difficult anorectal fistula: a prospective study. Dis Colon Rectum 2007;50: 2168–72.

25. Christoforidis D, Etzioni DA, Goldberg SM, et al. Treatment of complex anal fistulas with the collagen fistula plug. Dis Colon Rectum 2008;51:1482–7.

26. Lawes DA, Efron JE, Abbas M, et al. Early experience with the bioabsorbable anal fistula plug. World J Surg 2008;32:1157–9.

27. Thekkinkattil D, Botterill I, Ambrose S, et al. Efficacy of the anal fistula plug in complex anorectal fistulae. Colorectal Dis 2008 Jul 15; [Epub].

28. Fine AP. Laparoscopic repair of inguinal hernia using Surgisis mesh and fibrin sealant. JSLS 2006; 10:461–5.

29. Edelman DS, Selesnick H. "Sports" hernia: treatment with biologic mesh (Surgisis). A preliminary study. Surg Endosc 2006;20:971–3.

30. Catena F, Ansaloni L, Leone A, et al. Lichtenstein repair of inguinal hernia with Surgisis inguinal hernia matrix soft-tissue graft in immunodepressed patients. Hernia 2005;9:29–31.

31. Oelschlager BK, Pellegrini CA, Hunter J, et al. Biologic prosthesis reduces recurrence after laparoscopic paraesophageal hernia repair. Ann Surg 2006;244:481–90.

32. Helton WS, Fisichella PM, Berger R, et al. Short-term outcomes with small intestinal submucosa for ventral abdominal hernia. Arch Surg 2005;140:549–62.

33. Breunig KH, Warren SM. Immediate bilateral breast reconstruction with implants and inferolateral AlloDerm slings. Ann Plast Surg 2005;55:232–9.

34. Sampaio Goes JC. Periareolar mammoplasty: double-skin technique with application of polyglactine or mixed mesh. Plast Reconstr Surg 1996;97: 959–68.

35. Sampaio Goes JC. Periareolar mammoplasty: double-skin technique with application of mesh support. Clin Plast Surg 2002;29:349–64.

36. Seymour PE, Leventhal DD, Pribitkin EA. Lip augmentation with porcine small intestinal submucosa. Arch Facial Plast Surg 2008;10:30–3.

Laser-Assisted Liposuction

Alberto Goldman, MD[a,*], Robert H. Gotkin, MD, FACS[b]

KEYWORDS

- Laser lipolysis • Laser-assisted liposuction • Nd YAG laser

Over the past 30 years, liposuction has become an increasingly popular procedure. According to the American Society for Aesthetic Plastic Surgery, liposuction has been the most commonly performed cosmetic surgical procedure every year of this decade.[1] From its modern reinvention over 30 years ago, in which large uterine curettes and gynecologic aspirators were used to remove fat,[2,3] to the myriad technological advances that exist today, liposuction has undergone many changes. These changes can be divided into three main categories: changes in anesthesia management, changes in equipment and cannula size, and changes in the actual methods of treating and removing fat.

In the 1980s, liposuction usually was performed as a hospital inpatient procedure under general anesthesia, and it often required transfusion of autologous blood to replace that which was lost during the procedure. In 1988, Klein[4] published his landmark article on the tumescent technique; this method of administering large quantities of very dilute buffered lidocaine and epinephrine significantly reduced intraoperative blood loss and allowed the procedure to be moved from an inpatient setting to an office or other outpatient setting. Although slow to be adopted by many plastic surgeons, when properly used, Klein's tumescent technique dramatically improved the safety of liposuction and became incorporated into the procedure.[5]

The dramatic reduction in intraoperative blood loss and postoperative ecchymoses improved the recovery for patients undergoing liposuction. Surgeons continued to refine the procedure with the addition of internal ultrasound-assisted liposuction,[6-8] external ultrasound-assisted lipoplasty,[9] and power-assisted lipoplasty.[10] Parallel to these developments, Apfelberg[11-13] was beginning to study laser-assisted liposuction; this preliminary investigation utilized a YAG optical fiber contained within a liposuction cannula. The investigators concluded that no clear benefit was demonstrated with the laser; the US Food and Drug Administration (FDA) did not approve the technique, and the sponsoring laser company did not pursue the study. In the late 1990s, Neira and colleagues began studying the effects of low-level laser on adipose tissue.[14-17] At the same time, Blugerman[18] and Blugerman, Schavelzon, and Goldman[19-21] were using 1064 nm neodymium:yttrium-aluminum-garnet (Nd:YAG) laser energy, conducted by means of an optical fiber, within a 1 mm introducer cannula, in direct contact with adipose tissue. They found that the energy from the laser resulted in adipocyte lysis and other salutary side effects of the procedure and patient recovery. Badin and colleagues[22,23] arrived at very similar findings: less intraoperative blood loss, less postoperative ecchymoses, and improved skin tightening and skin redraping during the recovery process.

These findings have spurred a tremendous interest in laser lipolysis and laser-assisted liposuction. With the broad approval by the FDA in October 2006, of a 1064 nm Nd:YAG laser (Smartlipo, Cynosure, Incorporated, Westford, Massachusetts) for surgical incision, excision, vaporization, ablation and coagulation in soft tissues, and laser lipolysis, this interest has become even more magnified. Other lasers also have received FDA approval in the United States, and it appears that

The authors have no significant financial interest in any of the companies mentioned herein.
[a] Clinica Goldman of Plastic Surgery, Av. Augusto Meyer 163 Conj. 1203, Porto Alegre, RS, Brazil 90550-110
[b] Cosmetique Dermatology, Laser & Plastic Surgery, LLP, 625 Park Avenue, New York, NY 10065, USA
* Corresponding author.
E-mail address: alberto@goldman.com.br (A. Goldman).

Clin Plastic Surg 36 (2009) 241–253
doi:10.1016/j.cps.2008.11.005
0094-1298/08/$ – see front matter © 2009 Elsevier Inc. All rights reserved.

laser-assisted liposuction, although just one of many tools in the armamentarium of the aesthetic surgeon performing body contouring, has emerged as a hot technique in aesthetic plastic surgery.

SCIENCE

The laser–tissue interaction in adipose tissue has been described by many investigators.[11–28] Whether the laser acts directly upon the fat[18–25] or whether it is administered transcutaneously,[14–17] the final common pathway appears to be similar. Neira,[14–17] Goldman,[24] Ichikawa,[25] and their respective colleagues have elucidated this.

Neira's technique involved the external, transcutaneous application of low-level laser energy using a 635 nm diode laser with a maximum power of 10 mW. Even at these low energy delivery levels, Neira found a time- and, therefore, dose-dependent effect of laser energy on adipocytes. This was contrasted with a control population that received only tumescent solution without exposure to laser energy. At exposure times of 4 minutes, there was partial disruption of about 80% of the adipocytes' cell membranes. At longer exposure times (6 minutes), there was almost complete disruption in 99% of adipocyte cell membranes. In addition to this lipolysis, the laser energy also appeared to disrupt adipose connective tissue. In the control group, there was no change in the size, shape, or integrity of the adipocytes. With the spillage of intracellular contents into the extracellular or interstitial space, there was easier fat extraction, a reduction in surgical trauma, and a more abbreviated postoperative recovery.

Although these findings could not be confirmed independently by Brown and colleagues,[26]

Ichikawa and colleagues[25] subsequently showed the histologic findings in fat subjected to direct treatment with the 1064 nm Nd:YAG laser. In both photomicroscopic and scanning electron microscopic studies, Ichikawa demonstrated greater destruction of human adipocytes in laser-irradiated fat compared with nonlaser-irradiated controls. There seemed to be a dose-dependent degeneration of adipocyte cell membranes, vaporization and liquefaction of fat cells, and collagen fiber coagulation in response to the 1064 nm Nd:YAG laser irradiation.

With an Nd:YAG laser in direct contact with adipose tissue, Goldman[20,24] and Badin[22,23] demonstrated adipocyte cell membrane rupture, coagulation of small vessels within the adipose tissue, coagulation of adipose and dermal collagen, and a reorganization of the reticular dermis (**Fig. 1, 2**). The latter is associated with a process of neocollagenesis in the deep dermis and the dermal fat junction. These histologic findings seem to correlate with the clinical findings of a reduction in intraoperative blood loss, reduction in postoperative ecchymoses, a more comfortable postoperative recovery, a rapid return to activities of daily living (ADL), and enhanced skin tightening and skin redraping as a result of the neocollagenesis.

Kim and Geronemus[27] also confirmed similar findings; the lipolysis produced by the Nd:YAG laser acting in adipose tissue is an elegant and minimally invasive option associated with demonstrable reduction in fat volume, irrespective of subject weight change. There was excellent patient tolerance and the benefit of dermal tightening. The postoperative recovery was quick, and patients had a rapid return to ADL. MRI studies performed before and 3 months following surgery showed an average 17% reduction in

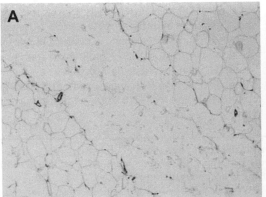 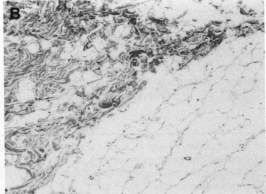

Fig. 1. (*A*) Laser-induced lipolysis (H & E: 40×). (*B*) Laser-induced lipolysis and adipose collagen coagulation (H & E: 40×).

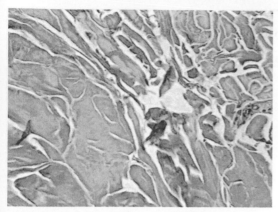

Fig. 2. Collagen coagulation (H & E: 100×).

adipose tissue volume in the areas treated; site-specific analysis revealed a 25% reduction in the submental area and an overall 14% reduction in the trunk and extremities.

Mordon and colleagues,[28] also demonstrated similar clinical and histologic findings using a continuous-wave 980 nm diode laser (Pharaon [Osyris; Hellemmes, France] and Lipotherme [Med-Surge Advances, Dallas, Texas]). At similar power settings as the pulsed Nd:YAG, the histologic findings were similar. This laser has the capability of higher wattage than the Nd:YAG laser; however, at these higher powers, there was carbonization noted in the adipose tissue and collagen fibers. This is significant, because carbonization and charring of tissues is much more likely to lead to unfavorable and unacceptable scarring internally and possibly externally. Perhaps the different pulse profile may be responsible for this; the continuous-wave diode and the pulsed Nd:YAG interact with adipose tissue in a different manner. The continuous waveform is more likely to char the tissues than a high peak power, but short duration pulsed waveform. The latter is more in harmony with the thermal relaxation time of the tissues.

The mechanism of action on a cellular level is caused by a specific laser–tissue interaction that is defined by the process of selective photothermolysis;[29] some features of this interaction are wavelength-dependent, and some are independent of wavelength used. There are three wavelengths currently on the market in the United States for laser lipolysis: pulsed 1064 nm, pulsed 1320 nm, and CW 980 nm diode. All three wavelengths generate infrared light energy that is absorbed by adipocytes and converted to heat. This absorption of energy causes deformation of the adipocyte, volume expansion and, subsequently, cell rupture. The adipocytes exposed to the highest energies undergo a photoacoustic or

photomechanical disruption; those exposed to lower energies (further from the tip of the optical fiber) undergo a photothermal change. The latter results in cellular deformation and expansion, but may not lead to immediate rupture; because of the changes in membrane permeability, however, many of these cells eventually die. The cellular debris is metabolized, and the metabolic by-products are excreted by means of the liver or kidneys. An additional effect of the laser-induced heating of the tissues appears to be a photostimulatory effect; this phenomenon is a lower energy process that occurs even further from the fiber tip and has broad overall activity on dermal and adipose collagen.

The 1064 nm wavelength also is known to be absorbed by oxyhemoglobin, and has even better absorption by methemoglobin (**Fig. 2**). Because of these absorption characteristics, this wavelength is effective in coagulating small blood vessels within the fat and seems to be responsible for the histologic and clinical findings noted by several investigators.[18–25]

As of June 2008, there were four devices approved by the FDA for laser lipolysis in the United States (**Table 1**). The pulsed 1064 nm Nd:YAG laser (Smartlipo [Cynosure; DEKA, Calenzano, Italy]) used for laser lipolysis has a pulse width of 100 milliseconds; the default energy delivery is 150 mJ/pulse and 40 Hz, but the energy per pulse and the pulses per second settings are variable. The original laser marketed in the United States and internationally had a maximum power of 6 W; this has been increased to 18 W as a stand-alone 1064 nm Nd:YAG laser. Cynosure now also markets a 1064 nm and 1320 nm multiplexed system with a maximum of 20 watts at 1064 nm and 12 W at 1320 nm. The 1064 nm pulse width is 150 milliseconds, and the 1320 nm pulse width is 212 milliseconds. Either wavelength can be used alone, or the two can be used together in a multiplexed fashion. The original 6 W laser came with an optical fiber of 300 μm in diameter; a 600 μm diameter fiber is also available. Both can be passed through a 1 mm microcannula; however the 600 μm fiber passes more easily through a 1.5 mm external diameter microcannula. The larger fiber and the larger microcannula, and the higher-powered lasers, are more robust and efficient for lipolysis.

The different absorption characteristics of the 1064 nm and 1320 nm wavelengths are responsible for their distinctive actions in adipose tissue. As noted in **Fig. 3**, the 1320 nm wavelength has a higher coefficient of absorption in water than the 1064 nm wavelength. In adipose tissue, this wavelength is strongly absorbed with less

Table 1
Lasers approved by the US Food and Drug Administration for laser lipolysis as of June 2008

	Smartlipo	Smartlipo-MPX	CoolLipo	LipoLite	Lipotherme
Manufacturer	Cynosure	Cynosure	CoolTouch	Syneron	Osyris/Med Surge Advances
Wavelength (nm)	1064	1064, 1320	1320	1064	980 diode
Maximum power (watts)	18	20, 12	15	?	25
Pulse width (μsec)	100	150	100	100–800	(CW)
Fiber size (s) (μm)	300, 600	600	200, 320, 500	550	600
Repetition rate	40	40	20–50	50	N/A
Pulse energy (mJ)	150	500, 300	?	<250–800	N/A

scattering compared with the 1064 nm wavelength. Therefore, the 1320 nm wavelength is extremely effective at rapidly heating adipose tissue in a very localized manner; most of the energy is absorbed in a small region immediately around the tip of the optical fiber. This is in contrast to the 1064 nm wavelength, in which energy diffuses over a broader treatment area, with a more controlled temperature elevation, more generalized heating of the fat, and better activity in hemoglobin. With water as the target chromophore of the 1320 nm wavelength, there is also a much greater effect on dermal collagen; this results in improved collagen shrinkage and skin tightening.

CoolTouch (Roseville, California) markets a 1320 nm Nd:YAG laser for laser lipolysis (CoolLipo). This pulsed Nd:YAG also has a pulse width of 100 milliseconds, power up to 15 W and a repetition of 20 to 50 Hz. Available optical fibers are 200, 320, and 500 μm in diameter. This device received FDA approval for laser-assisted lipolysis in January 2008.

Syneron (Yokneam, Israel) received FDA clearance for laser lipolysis for its entry into the laser-assisted liposuction market (LipoLite) in May 2008. This laser is also a pulsed 1064 nm Nd:YAG, but features a variable pulse width (100 to 800 milliseconds) and variable pulse energy (less than 250 to 800 mJ per pulse). It fires up to 50 Hz, but the power is not specified.

The other device currently available in the United States for direct internal interaction with adipose tissue is the 980 nm diode laser

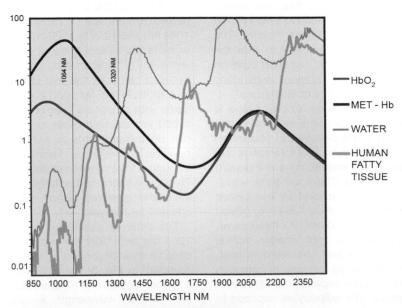

Fig. 3. Coefficients of absorption of water and human fatty tissue.

(Lipotherme [MedSurge Advances, Dallas, Texas]).[28] Other companies have similar devices in their pipelines, but are awaiting FDA clearance. Because the 1064 nm Nd:YAG laser has been available in the United States and FDA-approved for the longest period of time compared with the other devices, it is the most studied regarding its clinical and histological effects and has the most prior publications.

Studies on the thermal energy generated in laser lipolysis are beginning to reveal important information on correlations between skin surface temperature and skin shrinkage or contraction. Patients undergoing laser lipolysis had tattoos placed to mark the abdominal and thigh skin in 5 cm square areas. The laser lipolysis was conducted with a multiplexed device emitting 1064 nm energy at 20 watts and 1320 nm energy at 12 watts. The procedure was performed in order to obtain the usual clinical endpoints for aesthetically pleasing body contouring. The square areas were measured at 3 months and revealed an average 18% contraction (Barry DiBernardo, MD and Bruce Katz, MD, personal communication, June, 2008). In the authors' opinion, this contraction is likely to increase somewhat over the next 3 months, as the clinical end point in the healing process has not been reached.

In addition, the optimal skin surface temperature necessary in order to obtain maximal skin contraction, without carbonization or excessive thermal injury, is being studied. It appears that this optimum temperature is between 35° and 40°C. With the tip of the optical fiber 5 mm below the skin surface, the maximum skin surface temperature before tissue necrosis noted is 47°C (Bruce Katz, MD, personal communication, 2008). These types of data are very important in order to obtain the best possible clinical results and to define the safety limits of the procedure. As more devices with more power enter the marketplace, the latter is crucial.

INDICATIONS, CONTRAINDICATIONS, AND PATIENT SELECTION

The main indication for the use of laser lipolysis and laser-assisted liposuction is body contouring. It can be used for primary and secondary procedures; it is useful for small, well-defined, localized accumulations of excess fat or for larger areas of body contouring. As with any lipoplasty technique, laser-assisted liposuction is used best in patients who are at or near their ideal body weight, who have realistic expectations and have localized collections of excess adipose tissue. In essence, any patient who is a candidate for traditional liposuction is a candidate for laser-assisted liposuction.

The field of candidates expands over that of traditional liposuction, however, because laser-assisted liposuction is better able to treat some of those patients with skin laxity that would not have acceptable skin redraping with traditional techniques. Laser lipolysis also can be used to treat lipomas, gynecomastia, axillary hyperhidrosis,[30,31] and interstitial fluid malar pouches; it can be used to refine and contour flaps and to treat cellulite.[32]

Similar to traditional liposuction, contraindications to laser-assisted liposuction are unrealistic expectations on the part of the patient, pregnancy or lactation, allergy to lidocaine, and any general medical issues that would prevent someone from being able to have local anesthesia. If the procedure is to be performed under intravenous sedation, epidural block or general anesthesia (usually because of being combined with other procedures) the patient must be in good general medical condition to undergo such anesthetic management. The authors have found no procedure-specific contraindications to laser-assisted liposuction.

In selecting appropriate patients for this procedure, the surgeon should apply many of the dictums that apply to traditional liposuction. The preoperative consultation should include an evaluation of the patient's goals and expectations. If the procedure is being performed for purposes of body contouring, the areas of accumulation of excess fat should be delineated; the quality, thickness, turgor, and elasticity of the overlying skin should be determined. The pinch test, an important maneuver for any experienced liposuction surgeon, should be employed preoperatively to evaluate skin thickness, skin elasticity, and adipose thickness; intraoperatively to monitor the progress of the procedure; and postoperatively to evaluate the quality of the result.

If the laser is being utilized to treat axillary hyperhidrosis, it is helpful to employ a starch–iodine test preoperatively in order to precisely define the areas of greatest sweat production. This should be performed, photographed, measured, and compared with the postoperative result. When laser lipolysis is used to treat gynecomastia or to thin or contour a flap, there is essentially no difference in the preoperative evaluation or patient selection compared with traditional liposuction.

If laser lipolysis is being employed to treat cellulite, not only are the areas of cellulite important to evaluate preoperatively, but other areas that may benefit from body contouring need to be examined also. The importance here lies in the potential donor sites for autologous fat transplantation; this donor fat must be harvested with traditional liposuction—not with laser-assisted liposuction—

so as to maintain the integrity and viability of the adipocytes for transplantation.[32,33] Autologous fat is very useful to enhance the deepest, most concave areas of contour deformity in the correction of cellulite.

TECHNIQUE

Laser-assisted liposuction may be performed under local anesthesia alone, or supplemented with intravenous sedation, epidural block, or general anesthesia. This is an individual choice between the surgeon and the patient. Irrespective of anesthetic choice, the patient is marked in the standing position. If treatment is for cellulite, it is helpful to use various markers of different colors in order to mark areas of elevation and depression.[32] Once marked, the patient is brought to the operating room and prepped circumferentially in the standing position.[33] Following the preparation, the patient is placed on the operating table upon sterile drapes; this will allow the patient to be turned during the procedure without having to re-prep.[34,35] A single intravenous dose of a first-generation cephalosporin usually is administered.

If the procedure is expected to last 1 hour or more, external pneumatic compression devices (eg, Venodyne, Columbus, Mississippi) are placed on the legs, and the patient is sedated if desired. Subcutaneous infiltration of warmed Klein's tumescent solution, or some similar solution combining buffered lidocaine and epinephrine, precedes laser application to the areas of unwanted fat. Klein's solution contains 500 mg lidocaine, 1 mg epinephrine and 12.5 cc of 8.4% $NaHCO_3$ per liter of normal saline. This makes a buffered solution containing approximately 0.05% lidocaine, 1:1,000,000 units epinephrine. The total volume of subcutaneous infiltration depends upon surgeon preference and the overall size of the treatment area. The solution is warmed to minimize any discomfort associated with a temperature difference between the tissue and the fluid. Warming also helps to maintain core body temperature. The procedure is initiated following a 10- to 20-minute delay to allow for appropriate diffusion of the fluid and adequate vasoconstriction. Neira[15] compared longer laser energy exposure times in the absence of tumescent solution with shorter exposure times in the presence of tumescent solution. His histologic findings were comparable in the two groups, and he concluded that the tumescent solution enhanced the laser's activity on adipocytes.

Direct laser application into the adipose tissue occurs by means of an optical fiber. This fiber (200 to 600 μm in diameter) is conducted within a stainless steel microcannula of 1 to 1.5 mm external diameter. An important distinction between the current laser-assisted liposuction and that investigated by Apfelberg[11–13] in the 1990s is the location of the tip of the optical fiber. In Apfelberg's study, the tip of the fiber was within the liposuction cannula so that only that fat that had been avulsed already by the suction was exposed to the activity of the laser. All current systems work by having the tip of the fiber extend beyond the end of the cannula by 2 to 3 mm. This 2 to 3 mm extension enables the direct activity of laser energy within the adipose tissue. The optical fiber is conducted by means of very fine, small-diameter instruments, and no high negative pressure suction occurs. Lipolysis and small vessel and collagen coagulation occur directly by means of the activity of the laser. This distinction has further importance relative to the minimally invasive nature of the procedure.

The optical fiber conducts both the therapeutic infrared light (980, 1064, or 1320 nm) and a helium–neon aiming beam (634 nm). The transillumination of the HeNe beam allows for precise localization of the fiber tip so that the surgeon is constantly aware of the location of laser activity. The intensity of the aiming beam is also clinically relevant. The brighter the intensity of the beam, the more superficial within the tissue the fiber tip is located. Conversely, a lower intensity transillumination of the HeNe beam means that the tip of the fiber is deeper in the tissues.

Other delivery systems are beginning to enter the marketplace. The two most significant new delivery systems are a combination laser application–suction cannula (CoolTouch) and a motion-sensing feedback hand piece (Cynosure). The former combines simultaneous aspiration with laser application by enclosing the fiber in a small-diameter suction cannula; this cannula has a Y shape at the proximal end to accommodate the entry of the fiber and the connection for aspiration tubing. Other manufacturers are developing similar delivery systems.

Cynosure's SmartSense hand piece contains a motion-sensing feedback chip that feeds back information on the movement of the cannula to the laser device; this enables the laser to shut down energy delivery if it senses cessation of cannula movement. This safety feature helps to prevent overaccumulation of thermal energy in a given area and, therefore, helps to prevent carbonization, burns, and consequent adverse scarring.

The duration of laser activity in the tissues is highly variable and depends upon the overall size of the treatment area, the thickness and volume

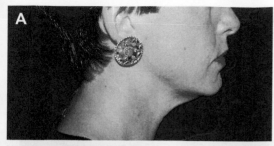

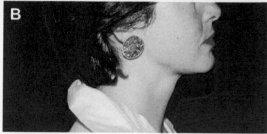

Fig. 4. 44-year-old woman is shown before (A) and 6 months after (B) laser-assisted liposuction of the neck.

of fat being removed, the degree of skin laxity, and the presence of previous internal scarring (eg, a secondary procedure). The surgeon senses a diminishing resistance to cannula movement as the procedure progresses. This indicates lipolysis and the presence of more liquefied fat (lysate) and less normal, untreated fat. As mentioned previously, the pinch test is another important factor in determining the clinical end point of treatment.

The resultant product of laser-assisted lipolysis is an oily lysate containing ruptured adipocytes and cellular debris mixed with tumescent solution. Aspiration of this lysate is the surgeon's choice. If the surgeon chooses to remove the mixture, it is removed by gentle aspiration using a 2 mm or 3 mm external diameter cannula and a negative

pressure of 0.3 to 0.5 atm (less than 50 kPa or 350 mm Hg). In this way, the minimally invasive nature of the procedure is preserved; high negative pressure suction that is traumatic to the tissues is avoided, and the postoperative recovery period is enhanced. It is the authors' experience that very small areas of treatment with low volumes of lysate do well without aspiration. This may be the case, for example, in the treatment of the anterior cervical area. In situations when minimal lipolysis is desired, and the laser is being used mainly for the photostimulatory effect of collagen contraction, here, too, it may not be necessary to aspirate. This latter example often applies to the treatment of cellulite.

Hemoglobin, hematocrit, serum cholesterol, and serum triglycerides were measured in 20 patients in the preoperative period and 1 day, 1 week and 1 month following laser-assisted liposuction. No significant changes were noted.[20]

Following surgery, the use of compression garments is, again, the individual surgeon's choice. As long as they are not too constrictive, the garments are usually helpful in reducing edema and improving skin redraping. During the first 1 to 2 weeks following the procedure, the patient may be started on a postoperative physiotherapeutic routine to hasten the resolution of edema. Devices such as the Tri-Active (Cynosure), Endermologie (LPG; Cedex, France), VelaShape or VelaSmooth (Syneron) may be employed.

RESULTS

Laser lipolysis and laser-assisted liposuction have proven to be safe and effective methods of body contouring. Although the early clinical results may be similar to those obtained by traditional liposuction, the histologic findings suggest explanations for the differences being seen in the

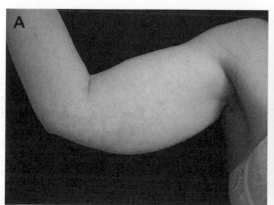

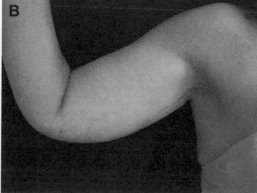

Fig. 5. 54-year-old woman is shown before (A) and 8 months after (B) laser-assisted liposuction of the arms.

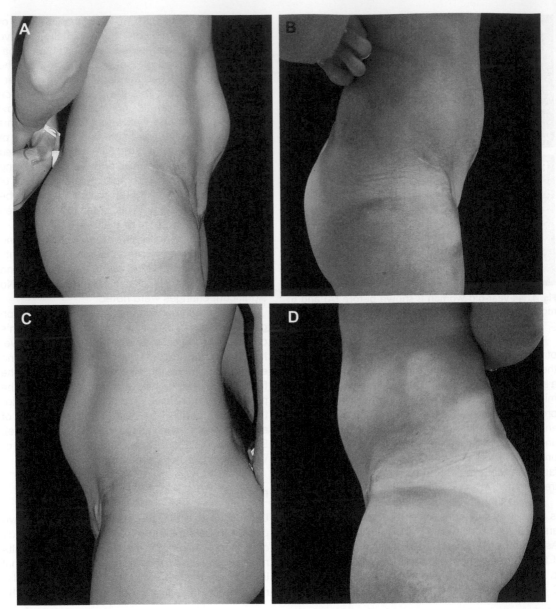

Fig. 6. 26-year-old woman is shown before (*A, C*) and 6 months after (*B, D*) laser-assisted liposuction of the abdomen.

clinical course of recovery and the final clinical result. The coagulation of blood vessels noted histologically correlates with the reduction in peri-operative and postoperative bleeding and ecchymoses. The coagulation of collagen in the adipose tissue and the deep dermis, associated with neocollagenesis and reorganization of the reticular dermis, explains the skin contraction or shrinkage noted in the later postoperative course. This capacity of the laser to produce skin contraction is very important in the treatment of patients with some degree of skin laxity who may not be candidates for traditional liposuction (**Figs. 4–10**).

Like traditional liposuction, laser-assisted liposuction is useful in combination with other surgical procedures such as facelift, abdominoplasty, thighplasty, reduction mammaplasty, and breast reconstruction. In the absence of platysmal banding, when used in the neck, laser-assisted liposuction

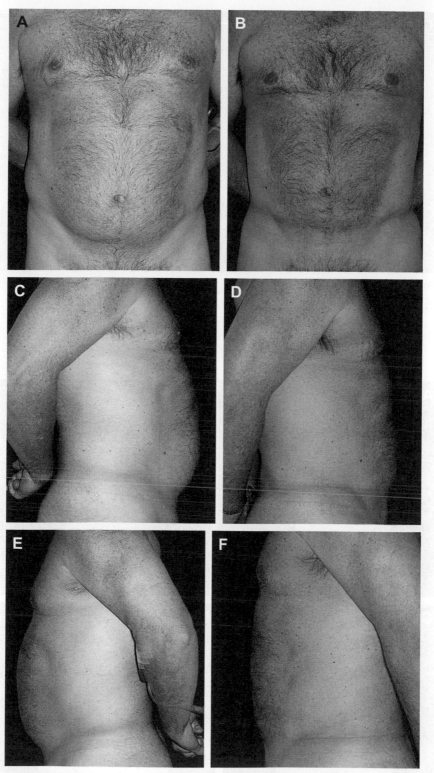

Fig. 7. 47-year-old man before (*A, C, E, G*) and 6 months after (*B, D, F, H*) laser-assisted liposuction of the abdomen, hips, and flanks.

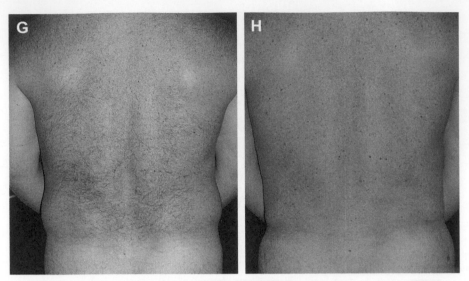

Fig. 7. (continued)

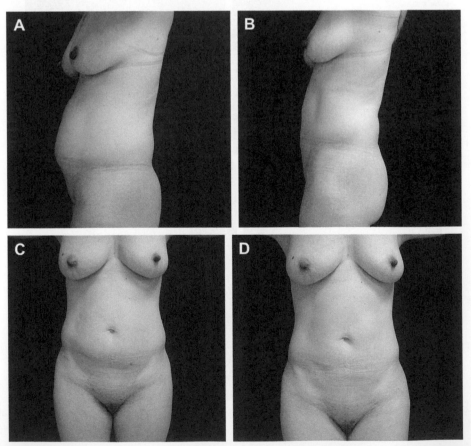

Fig. 8. 38-year-old woman is shown before (*A*, *C*) and 6 months after (*B*, *D*) laser-assisted liposuction of the abdomen, hips, and flanks.

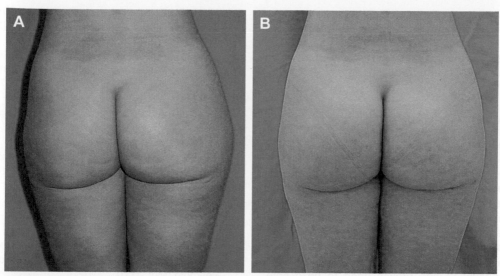

Fig. 9. 32-year-old woman is shown before (*A*) and 6 months after (*B*) laser-assisted liposuction of hips and thighs for treatment of cellulite.

may preclude having to open the neck in a facelift. In the surgical body-contouring procedures, it is helpful to contour the peripheral or adjacent areas not directly affected by dermatolipectomy.

COMPLICATIONS

Side effects and complications of laser-assisted liposuction are rare, and most do not appear to be specific for the use of the laser. The exception is thermal injury. The energy produced at the fiber tip can build up to harmful and damaging levels

rather promptly if the surgeon's attention is diverted. Excessive subcutaneous or cutaneous thermal injury can occur. Any other potential complication or side effect noted with traditional liposuction can occur with laser-assisted liposuction also. There will be minimal ecchymoses, some edema, and the usual cutaneous anesthesia noted following traditional liposuction. When laser treatment is very superficial—in order to obtain maximal skin contraction or in the treatment of cellulite—the cutaneous anesthesia may last somewhat longer.[32] Similar to traditional

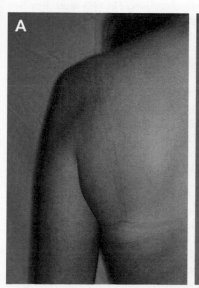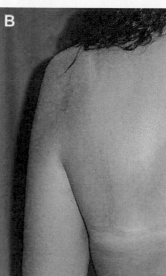

Fig. 10. 28-year-old woman is shown before (*A*) and 6 months after (*B*) laser-assisted liposuction of the posterior axillary area.

liposuction, minor aesthetic differences or asymmetries are the most common complication. As more powerful devices populate the market, greater care will have to be exercised to avoid thermal injuries.

SUMMARY

The ongoing search for new tools and alternative techniques in liposuction is related to an underlying desire of surgeons to improve the safety of the technique, reduce the downtime for patients, and enhance the ultimate cosmetic result. By reducing blood loss, minimizing both aesthetic and anesthetic side effects and complications, and by promoting improvements in skin contraction and redraping following surgery, laser-assisted liposuction has proven itself to be a safe, effective, and useful addition to the armamentarium of the plastic surgeon performing body contouring. A growing body of experience and evidence indicates that the technique can expand the base of patients who are candidates for primary liposuction as well as those who desire secondary procedures. The fact that this small-caliber, minimally invasive technology can be utilized very superficially, without leaving a footprint in the tissue, while coagulating collagen, inducing neocollagenesis and the accompanying skin contraction, is a tremendous advantage to surgeon and patient.

REFERENCES

1. Annual Cosmetic Surgery National Data Bank Statistics, American Society for Aesthetic Plastic Surgery, 2000–2007.
2. Kesselring UK. Regional fat aspiration for body contouring. Plast Reconstr Surg 1983;72(5):610–9.
3. Kesselring UK, Meyer R. A suction curette for removal of excessive local deposits of subcutaneous fat. Plast Reconstr Surg 1978;62(2):305–6.
4. Klein JA. Anesthesia for liposuction in dermatologic surgery. J Dermatol Surg Oncol 1988;14(10): 1124–32.
5. Klein JA. Tumescent technique for local anesthesia improves safety in large-volume liposuction. Plast Reconstr Surg 1993;92(6):1085–98.
6. Zocchi ML. Ultrasonic liposculpturing. Aesthetic Plast Surg 1992;16:287–98.
7. Maxwell GP, Gingrass MK. Ultrasound-assisted lipoplasty: a clinical study of 250 consecutive patients. Plast Reconstr Surg 1998;101(1):189–202.
8. Zocchi ML. Ultrasonic-assisted lipectomy. Adv Plast Reconstr Surg 1995;11:197–221.
9. Silberg BN. The technique of external ultrasound-assisted lipoplasty. Plast Reconstr Surg 1998;101(2): 552.
10. Fodor PB, Vogt PA. Power-assisted lipoplasty (PAL): a clinical pilot study comparing PAL to traditional lipoplasty (TL). Aesthetic Plast Surg 1999;23(6):379–85.
11. Apfelberg DB. Laser-assisted liposuction may benefit surgeons, patients. Clin Laser Mon 1992; 10(12):193–4.
12. Apfelberg DB, Rosenthal S, Hunsted JP, et al. Progress report on multicenter study of laser-assisted liposuction. Aesthetic Plast Surg 1994;18(3):259–64.
13. Apfelberg DB. Results of multicenter study of laser-assisted liposuction. Clin Plast Surg 1996;23(4): 713–9.
14. Neira R, Solarte E, Reyes MA, et al. Low-level laser-assisted lipoplasty: a new technique. In: Proceedings of the World Congress on Liposuction. Dearborn (MI): 2000.
15. Neira R, Arroyave J, Ramirez H, et al. Fat Liquefaction: effect of low-level laser energy on adipose tissue. Plast Reconstr Surg 2002;110(3):912–22.
16. Neira R, Ortiz-Neira C. Low-level laser-assisted liposculpture: clinical report of 700 cases. Aesthetic Plast Surg 2002;22(5):451–5.
17. Neira R, Toledo L, Arroyave J, et al. Low-level laser-assisted liposuction: the Neira 4L technique. Clin Plast Surg 2006;33(1):117–27.
18. Blugerman G. Laser lipolysis for the treatment of localized adiposity and cellulite. In: Abstracts of the World Congress on Liposuction. Dearborn (MI): 2000.
19. Schavelzon D, Blugerman G, Goldman A, et al. Laser lipolysis. In: Abstracts of the 10th International Symposium of Cosmetic Laser Surgery. Las Vegas (NV): 2001.
20. Goldman A, Schavelzon DE, Blugerman GS. Laser lipolysis: liposuction using Nd:YAG laser. Rev Soc Bras Cir Plast 2002;17(1):17–21.
21. Goldman A, Schavelzon D, Blugerman G. Liposuction using neodymium:yttrium-aluminum-garnet laser. International Abs. Plast Reconstr Surg 2003; 111(7):2497.
22. Badin AZD, Moraes LM, Gondek LB, et al. Laser lipolysis: flaccidity under control. Aesthetic Plast Surg 2002;26(5):335–9.
23. Badin AZD, Gondek LB, Garcia MJ, et al. Analysis of laser lipolysis effects on human tissue samples obtained from liposuction. Aesthetic Plast Surg 2005; 29(4):281–6.
24. Goldman A. Submental Nd:YAG laser-assisted liposuction. Lasers Surg Med 2006;38(3):181–4.
25. Ichikawa K, Miyasaka M, Tanaka R, et al. Histologic evaluation of the pulsed Nd:YAG laser for laser lipolysis. Lasers Surg Med 2005;36(1):43–6.
26. Brown SA, Rohrich RJ, Kenkel J, et al. Effect of low-level laser therapy on abdominal adipocytes before

lipoplasty procedures. Plast Reconstr Surg 2004; 113(6):1796–804.

27. Kim KH, Geronemus RG. Laser lipolysis using a novel 1064 nm Nd:YAG laser. Dermatol Surg 2006;32:241–8.

28. Mordon S, Eymard-Maurin AF, Wassmer B, et al. Histologic evaluation of laser lipolysis: pulsed 1064 nm Nd:YAG laser versus CW 980 nm diode laser. Aesthetic Surg J 2007;27(3):263–8.

29. Anderson RR, Parrish JA. Selective photothermolysis: precise microsurgery by selective absorption of pulsed radiation. Science 1983;220:524–7.

30. Wollina U, Goldman A, Berger U, et al. Esthetic and cosmetic dermatology. Dermatol Ther 2008;21:118–30.

31. Goldman A, Wollina U. Subdermal Nd-YAG laser for axillary hyperhidrosis. Dermatol Surg 2008;34:756–62.

32. Goldman A, Gotkin RH, Sarnoff DS, et al. Cellulite: a new treatment approach combining subdermal Nd:YAG laser lipolysis and autologous fat transplantation. Aesthetic Surg J 2008;28(6):656–62.

33. Teimourian B, Chajchir A, Gotkin RH, et al. Semi-liquid autologous fat transplantation. Adv Plast Reconstr Surg 1989;5:57–84.

34. Teimourian B, Gotkin RH. Contouring the midtrunk in overweight patients. Aesthetic Plast Surg 1989;13:145–53.

35. Teimourian B. Suction lipectomy and body sculpturing. St. Louis: C.V. Mosby Company; 1987.

Commentary on "Laser-Assisted Liposuction"

Rodrigo Neira, MD

During the past decade, in an era of remarkable advances in technology and cybernetics, surgeons have developed co-adjuvant tools for liposuction procedures that do not harm the patient. Before adopting any new technology, however, we must be sure the technique meets three essential criteria: that it does no harm, that it improves outcomes, and that it improves the quality and duration of patients' recovery. Less invasive surgical procedures result in less surgical trauma and decrease the physiologic inflammatory response.[1,2]

In their article, Drs. Goldman and Gotkin review the procedure called "laser-assisted liposuction." They claim that the "SmartLipo" laser reduces the patient's downtime after the procedure and enhances the ultimate cosmetic result. This liposuction technique, they say, reduces blood loss and minimizes the side effects of anesthetics and the complications related to the procedure. The technique also improves skin contraction and re-draping after surgery. Drs. Goldman and Gotkin conclude that surgeons can use this small-caliber, minimally invasive technology superficially, without leaving a "footprint" in the patient's tissue, while inducing neocollagenesis and skin contraction that greatly benefit the patient. What is uncertain from Drs. Goldman and Gotkin's article is the amount of fat that can be extracted with this technique and the amount of blood that is found in the supernatant when the procedure is done.

Because adipose cells are very fragile,[3] lipolysis can be done simply, with minimal trauma, using traditional procedures such as the cannula or with other procedures such as ultrasound and the application of internal or external lasers. The main goal of developing surgical co-adjuvant tools is not to provide an easy, faster way to remove fat but instead is to help the surgeon access places where the fat is difficult to remove, such as those surrounded by a large amount of connective tissue. The connective tissue and retinaculum cutis supply blood to the skin and flaps that keep the tissues alive. Because the cellular membrane of the adipose cell is very fragile, it is easy to rupture and destroy it. The goal of the surgical procedure is easy fat extraction, but it also must focus on destroying the connective tissue that surrounds the adipose cell.

When my colleagues and I[4,5] used transmission electron microscopy and scanning electron microscopy techniques to study adipose tissue, we found that it is surrounded by connective tissue in amounts that vary from one part of the body to another. This finding explains the difficulty that plastic surgeons have in removing fat from some parts of the body.

The two different laser techniques developed to assist liposuction, the Nd:YAG laser SmartLipo and low-level laser liposuction using the Neira 4L laser, work in completely different ways. The first is an internal beam laser; the other is an external beam laser. The main goal of the cold, external low-level laser Neira 4L technique is to minimize trauma to the adipose tissue, surgical trauma, and the inflammatory response. The use of this "cold" low-level laser decreases pain after the procedure, improves the healing process, shortens the recovery time after the procedure, and facilitates patients' rapid return to daily activities.[6]

In their article, Drs. Goldman and Gotkin suggest that the Nd:YAG laser, an internal thermal laser, has the same effect on the adipose tissue as the low-level laser, which is a noninvasive tool employing a different approach and technique. Drs. Goldman and Gotkin stress that the Nd:YAG laser induces lipolysis, simultaneously coagulating tiny blood vessels and stimulating dermal and subdermal neocollagenesis. This claim, however, does not seem to have been substantiated as yet by histologic or other noninvasive diagnostic techniques.

Neocollagenesis in the deep dermis and dermal–fat junction, which is activated by a single touch of liposuction cannula, would lead to significant skin tightening and skin redraping. Sometimes, however, depressions and irregularities

Department of Plastic, Maxillofacial, and Hand Surgery, Red Deer Regional Hospital, Red Deer, Alberta, Canada
E-mail address: Rodrigoneiramd@aol.com

Clin Plastic Surg 36 (2009) 255–256
doi:10.1016/j.cps.2009.01.001
0094-1298/09/$ – see front matter © 2009 Elsevier Inc. All rights reserved

caused by secondary contraction of the dermis and collagen can be prevented. It would be interesting to know what effect the internal laser has on the skin in the mid-range follow-up.

Since Gasparotti's[7] study of superficial liposuction in 1992, many concerns have been published about its undesirable outcomes, including irregularities, uneven surfaces, secondary skin retraction, subcutaneous fibrosis, and subcutaneous deformities. These poor results occurred because doctors started using techniques they learned about at meetings before they had received adequate formal training. This phenomenon presents a real challenge in the field of plastic surgery both for the surgeon performing the new technique and for the researcher who described the technique. We all want to do what is best for our patients, and our efforts will be deemed successful by our ultimate judges—our patients.

Drs. Goldman and Gotkin have presented preliminary data about the use of SmartLipo, which may indeed, as they claim, be a powerful tool for preventing secondary cicatrization and skin deformities after superficial liposuction. Plastic surgeons and other researchers are invited to analyze deeply and carefully this interesting information provided by SmartLipo and perhaps to ponder it until further studies support the claims made for this procedure.

Following this commentary are some questions that I have made to the authors of SmartLipo and their answers. Every effort a researcher makes to enhance the standard of care should serve to improve the patient's quality of life; this improvement is our ultimate goal as plastic and reconstructive surgeons.

REFERENCES

1. Medrado AR, Pugliese LS, Reis SR, et al. Influence of low level laser therapy on wound healing and its biological action upon myofibroblasts. Laser Surg Med 2003;32(3):239–44.
2. Gavish L, Asher Y, Becker Y, et al. Low level laser irradiation stimulates mitochondrial membrane potential and disperses subnuclear promyelocytic leukemia protein. Lasers Surg Med 2004;35(5). 369–76.
3. Monteiro R, de Castro PMST, Calhau C, et al. Adipocyte size and liability to cell death. Obes Surg 2006; 16(6):804–6.
4. Neira R, Toledo L, Arroyabe J, et al. low-level assisted liposuction: the Neira 4L technique. Clin Plast Surg 2006;33:117–27.
5. Neira R, Ortiz C. Low-level laser-assisted liposculpture: clinical report of 700 cases. Aesthet Surg J 2002;22(5):451–7.
6. Neira R, Arroyave J, Ramirez H, et al. Fat liquefaction effect from low level laser energy; a new technique. Plastic and Reconstructive Surgery Journal 2002; 110(3):912–22.
7. Gasparotti M. Superficial liposuction: a new application of the technique for aged and flaccid skin. Aesthetic Plast Surg 1992;16:141–53.

"Laser-Assisted Liposuction": Questions and Answers

Rodrigo Neira, MD[a],*, Alberto Goldman, MD[b],
Robert H. Gotkin, MD, FACS[c]

KEYWORDS

- Laser-assisted liposuction • Internal laser
- External laser • Lipolysis

The following questions were posed by Dr. Rodrigo Neira and answered by Drs. Alberto Goldman and Robert H. Gotkin, authors of "Laser-Assisted Liposuction."

QUESTION

"Primum Non Nocere"

AUTHOR'S RESPONSE

First, do no harm. Second, as Albert Einstein said, "We must open the mind to new ideas."

After 8 years of experience using laser-assisted liposuction, and based on the principles already described by the authors and many other colleagues, it is our opinion that this tool represents a safe and effective procedure. It is an alternative option and, as with any medical treatment, it can have bad results, complications, or side effects. It was already well described in "Laser-Assisted Liposuction."

QUESTION

The tumescent technique has eliminated bleeding almost completely. How important is it to control bleeding with the traditional techniques?

AUTHOR'S RESPONSE

The affirmation in the question and the technique described in "Laser-Assisted Liposuction" have no relationship. The tumescent technique is related to the quantity and type of anesthetic solution. In laser-assisted liposuction, it is possible to use any kind of anesthesia, including tumescent. The effect of the laser (coagulation) in small blood vessels is related to the target chromophore to be reached (oxyhemoglobin) and not to the type or amount of injected solution. On the other hand, the laser used in this technique is a 1064-nm Nd:YAG (or 1320 nm), which is highly absorbed by this chromophore.

QUESTION

How do the features of this laser lipolysis permit a fast, comfortable postoperative recovery and a rapid return to activities of daily living by increasing surgical and thermal trauma?

AUTHOR'S RESPONSE

The assertion that laser lipolysis permits a fast, comfortable postoperative recovery and a rapid return to activities of daily living is based on clinical experience and on histologic studies and scientific publications. Some positive aspects related to the characteristics of laser-assisted lipolysis (LAL) are the use of a small cannula (1 mm), the tunnels in fatty tissue related to the laser action, and the effect of the energy in the adipocytes leading to lipolysis. It means that it is possible to remove this less dense and oily solution using a less negative pressure (half atmosphere instead of 1 atmosphere in a regular liposuction). The net effect is less surgical trauma.

QUESTION

Is excellent skin redraping a result of laser-induced skin tightening? Are secondary cicatrization and delayed cicatrization increased with internal laser? Does laser-assisted liposuction increase the high

* Corresponding author.
E-mail address: rodrigoneiramd@aol.com (R. Neira).

Clin Plastic Surg 36 (2009) 257–260
doi:10.1016/j.cps.2008.12.002
0094-1298/08/$ – see front matter © 2009 Elsevier Inc. All rights reserved.

risk for deformities and irregularities in the long term?

AUTHOR'S RESPONSE

It depends on the intensity and length of time during which the surgeon delivers the energy. It is a well-known principle that the action of different types of energy, including the external diode laser, is able to stimulate new collagen production. In this technique, the laser beam is acting in direct contact with the dermis. As with any new surgical technique, it has a learning curve.

QUESTION

Is this technology less invasive than the tumescent and external beam laser procedures?

AUTHOR'S RESPONSE

It is a different approach, and the intention of our article was not to compare these options.

QUESTION

Does this technology have fewer side effects in the short term and the long term?

AUTHOR'S RESPONSE

It is not the intention of the manuscript to compare techniques but to describe the main characteristics of this new tool in body sculpturing. Side effects were described in the manuscript.

QUESTION

Does this technology increase free radicals by increasing surgical and thermal trauma?

AUTHOR'S RESPONSE

According to clinical data and many publications (see the reference list for "Laser-Assisted Liposuction"), no evidence of this exists. The authors suggest removing the oily solution from the body by gentle aspiration.

QUESTION

Does this technique help in the inflammatory process?

AUTHOR' RESPONSE

Different kinds of lasers (mainly low-level laser energy) are related to anti-inflammatory effect. Unfortunately, we do not have studies or evidence about this effect using LAL.

QUESTION

Is the recovery time shorter?

AUTHOR'S RESPONSE

This point is a part of the text. It is well explained in all details, showing the relationship with the laser effects in the fat and surrounding tissues and the quality of the recovery time.

QUESTION

Is the surgical procedure safer than traditional techniques?

AUTHOR'S RESPONSE

It is not the intention of the manuscript to compare techniques but to show another option in terms of lipoplastic procedures.

QUESTION

Is the new technique easier to perform?

AUTHOR'S RESPONSE

Yes, it is. However, as with all surgical techniques, it has a learning curve. On the other hand, it is important to know and to understand the principles of laser physics and laser–tissue interaction.

QUESTION

Is the new procedure cost effective?

AUTHOR'S RESPONSE

This question is not related to the scientific material sent for publication.

QUESTION

How long and steep is the learning curve for the new technique?

AUTHOR'S RESPONSE

It depends on the skill of the surgeon and how well the surgeon is able to understand and apply the laser principles.

QUESTION

How easy is it to deal with side effects and complications of the "neopathology" that has been born?

AUTHOR'S RESPONSE

"Neopathology" is a harsh word; the authors prefer "neobenefits" or "neoadvances."

Complications and side effects are part of any kind of medical technique. A good physician must be prepared to avoid, to treat, and to manage these kinds of difficulties. The potential complications of LAL were described exhaustively in the manuscript.

QUESTION

Does the new technique offer better results?

AUTHOR'S RESPONSE

It is not the intention of the manuscript to compare techniques but to show how LAL works. The authors do not claim that this technique produces better results. It is only an alternative option with specific characteristics that were well described in the manuscript.

QUESTION

Are the side effects easier to repair than those of traditional procedures?

AUTHOR'S RESPONSE

This question was already discussed.

QUESTION

Does this technique create colloidal protein degeneration by increasing the temperature of the adipose tissue?

AUTHOR'S RESPONSE

We do not know.

QUESTION

Have peripheral nerves been destroyed (burned) by the hot laser cannula and are anesthesia and neuropraxis on the skin increased with the new technique?

AUTHOR'S RESPONSE

As in any case of surgical trauma, a normal and temporary decrease in the sensitivity of the skin occurs for a few weeks. Some studies demonstrated that no anatomic alterations occur in the nerves using this laser with coherent parameters. This study used three different histologic colorations (see references in the manuscript).

QUESTION

Does the new technique increase postoperative pain or just burn the peripheral nerves?

AUTHOR'S RESPONSE

We did not use the terminology "burning the peripheral nerves" in our study. Again, all the positive and negative effects related to the technique were described in the text. In fact, our clinical experience has documented less postoperative pain in most patients.

QUESTION

During long-term follow-up, have the smoothness and irregularities on the skin improved with the new technique?

AUTHOR'S RESPONSE

Yes. A new manuscript about this topic was approved for publication in the *Aesthetic Surgery Journal*. The article will be published in an upcoming issue of the journal.

QUESTION

How easy is it to deal with the secondary and tertiary cicatrization process after burning fat is increased?

AUTHOR'S RESPONSE

This point was already discussed.

QUESTION

In the long term, are scar tissue and fibrotic tissue less prevalent than is seen with traditional techniques?

AUTHOR'S RESPONSE

We believe that any kind of surgical trauma (including traditional liposuction) leads to internal scarring. It was not the intention of the study to compare this potential trauma with the trauma caused by other techniques.

QUESTION

Are the hardness and smoothness of the skin better with the new technique?

AUTHOR'S RESPONSE

In our clinical experience they are, but no study has compared this new technique with more traditional ones.

QUESTION

Is the risk for skin necrosis lower with the new technique?

AUTHOR'S RESPONSE

If the surgeon uses any energy-assisted form of liposuction (internal ultrasound, external ultrasound, laser), the possibility of thermal injury or even necrosis is real. But it is also true that with good sense and care, and based on our experience, this occurrence is rare.

QUESTION

Are fluid collection and seromas decreased with the new technique?

AUTHOR'S RESPONSE

It is our opinion that the potential is the same. No clinical studies have compared the incidence of seromas or fluid collection caused by LAL with that caused by other techniques.

QUESTION

Are local and systemic infections increased by the surgical trauma, which increases the burn surface?

AUTHOR'S RESPONSE

The manuscript has no description of burned tissue. The effects related to the laser action are the thermal effect (heat, not burn) and mainly the mechanical effect (ie, the shock of the laser beam against the targets: adipocytes, glands, or dermis).

QUESTION

Is the immunologic system affected by local burn?

AUTHOR'S RESPONSE

We do not know.

QUESTION

Has multisystemic response been increased with the additional thermal trauma?

AUTHOR'S RESPONSE

Multisystemic response is probably not increased, but no study has yet demonstrated a relationship between thermal trauma and multisystem response.

Clinical Applications of Radiofrequency: Nonsurgical Skin Tightening (Thermage)

Darryl J. Hodgkinson, MBBS, FRCS (C), FACS, FACCS

KEYWORDS

- Radiofrequency • Thermage • Skin tightening
- ThermacoolNXT • Nonsurgical • Dermal heating

Monopolar radiofrequency delivered through cooled epidermis and superficial dermis has been used since 2003 to deliver heating to the deeper dermis, creating thermal damage, the healing of which, from myofibroblastic and fibroblastic activities, results in a discernible tightening of skin. Thermage (Thermage, Inc., Hayward, California) is the manufacturer of ThermaCool devices, which deliver the radiofrequency.

ThermaCool operates in the 6 MHz radiofrequency range. The depth of penetration of the radiofrequency, the depth of damage, and hence remodeling, depend on the type of tip used in the machine and the energy delivered by the machine through the tip.

All ThermaCool devices have three components: a generator, a cooler and a hand piece with a treatment tip. The generator supplies the radiofrequency and monitors through a display unit, the output current, output energy, number of treatments, duration of treatment, and impedance. The ThermaCoolNXT system is shown in **Fig. 1.**

A return pad is applied to the patient, allowing the generator to supply the monopolar radiofrequency in a closed circuit between the device and the patient. In all treatment areas, a temporary marking grid is applied so that the operator can place the treatment tip accurately for each radiofrequency pulse, patterning the delivery of the radiofrequency in such a way as to obtain the optimal delivery of radiofrequency over the entire treated area. **Fig. 2** shows a diagram of the marking grid applied to treatment area to aid in delivery of radiofrequency.

The mechanism of action of the radiofrequency on tissue is heat-generated by the tissues' natural resistance to the movement of electrons within the radiofrequency field (Ohm's law). Ohm's law states that energy in joules = I^2 x Z x t, where Z is impedance, I is the current in amperes, and t is time in seconds.

The initial response is an immediate thermally induced collagen denaturation with a subsequent collagen fiber contraction. In the newer deeper tips, which penetrate deeper into the dermis, the same thermally induced denaturation and contraction affect the fibrous septae, allowing a three-dimensional contraction of the tissue. This deep heat also promotes an increase in the blood flow in the capillaries, thus producing an increase in the metabolism in the fat layers. The normal inflammatory phase of healing followed by collagen remodeling results in long-term dermal tightening and contour changes in the treated area. The initial response of tightening seen clinically is not caused by avascular necrosis of fat but by the breakdown of the hydrogen bonds in the collagen chain causing shrinkage of the normal collagen structure.

CLINICAL AND EXPERIMENTAL DATA

The initial reports by Fitzpatrick and colleagues[1] involved a single pass of the periorbital region

I receive no royalties or commissions from Thermage. All patients have given their permission for utilization of photographs.
The Cosmetic & Restorative Surgery Clinic, Double Bay, Sydney, Australia
E-mail address: dr_hodgkinson@bigpond.com

Clin Plastic Surg 36 (2009) 261–268
doi:10.1016/j.cps.2008.11.006

plasticsurgery.theclinics.com

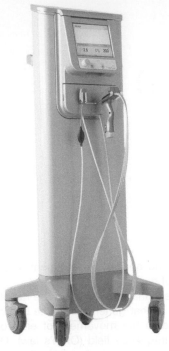

Fig. 1. ThermaCoolNXT machine. (*Courtesy of* Thermage, Inc., Hayward, CA; with permission.)

with a measurable increase in eyebrow elevation (62%) and improvement in the periorbital rhytids (83%) corresponding to patient satisfaction (similar rates). Abraham and colleagues[2] also noted brow elevation measured 12 weeks after treatment.

Fritz and colleagues[3] treated the nasolabial folds. The middle and lower face laxity was treated

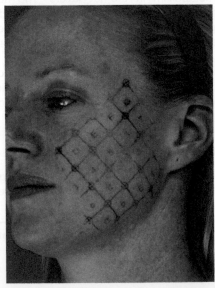

Fig. 2. Tattoo grid applied.

by Fritz and colleagues,[3] who noted that two radiofrequency treatments afforded a better result over a single treatment in the nasolabial fold. They also noted that significant improvement of the results occurred between 1 and 4 months after the procedure.

Koch,[4] from Stanford University, in a well-designed study, assessed the results of one and multiple treatments of radiofrequency on brow position and noted that 60% of patients had significant brow elevation with one treatment, and 80% of patients had significant elevation after four treatments. As early as 2004, their predictions were that other areas of the face and neck would respond well to radiofrequency and the clinical experience, and the development of new tips seems to support this.

Considering the jowl, Nahm and colleagues[5] treated one side only and noted a reduction in the jowl surface area of 22.6% compared with the nontreated area. Besides volumetric firming and lifting, other advantages noted in the skin have been the reduction of wrinkles and improvement of acne.[6,7]

The newest developments in Thermage delivery are multiple-pass techniques (staggering), keeping the tissues hot to give greater efficacy of the applied radiofrequency. Deeper tips, not to be used on the face, penetrate deeper into the skin for greater efficacy in body contouring and cellulite improvement.

TREATMENT TIPS

Treatment tips are one-time use only devices that deliver a fixed number of firings in a defined time range once the tip is activated. For sterility and quality purposes, the one-tip, one-patient, one-procedure process is established and inviolate. The range of tips in size, depth and penetration, and the number of firings has been expanded and as of this article, five different tips are available with multiple pulse configurations for each tip (**Fig 3**).

An appropriate tip for each anatomic area must be selected. The shallow-depth 0.5 cm ST tip is used for the eyelids. The shallow-depth ST 1.5^2 cm tip is used for the periorbital area, hands, and lips. The medium-depth tips 3^2 cm TC and STC tips are used for the face and neck. The newest deeper tip, DC, introduced in late 2007, is used for body contouring and replaces the previously used TC and STC tips for treating arms, thighs, abdomen, and buttocks. A cellulite tip, CL, with which I have not had experience, also was developed recently. **Fig. 4** shows the depth of penetration of the radiofrequency with different tip designs.

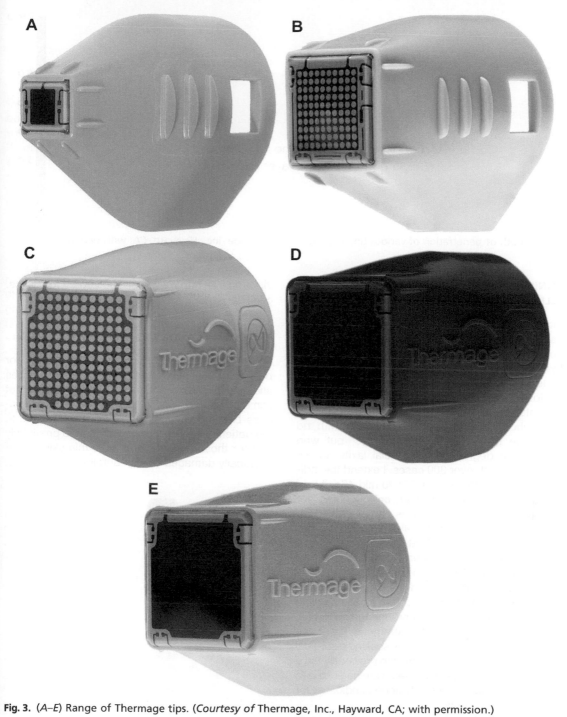

Fig. 3. (*A–E*) Range of Thermage tips. (*Courtesy of* Thermage, Inc., Hayward, CA; with permission.)

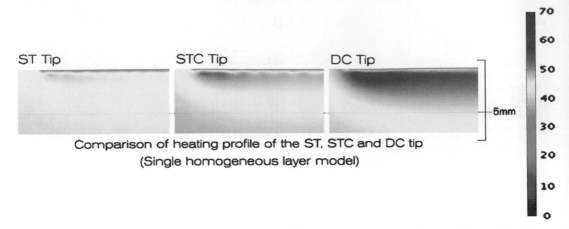

Fig. 4. Depth of penetration of various tips. (*Courtesy of* Thermage, Inc., Hayward, CA; with permission.)

CLINICAL APPLICATIONS, INCLUDING PATIENT SELECTION

Most experience, including my own over 3 years, has been in the face with tips designed to reduce periorbital rhytids—the 0.25^2 cm, and to firm in the submental and neck areas, cheeks, nasolabial folds, and jowl area—3^2 cm STC tip.

Most authors agree that the most appropriate patients or ideal patients are those in their mid-30s, who exhibit early signs of aging with no excessive rhytids or actinic damage[8] but who have some degree of early facial laxity. In my experience with over 300 cases, I extend the indications for patients in their 30s to mid-40s, if I regard them as realistic and only wishing for a modest improvement. Cases can be individualized, and an occasional well-maintained patient in her 50s can be a candidate.

If I can technically squeeze more than 2 cm of skin laxity, then I would not use Thermage, as the elevation of tissues is in the range of millimeters. Alternatively, if I consider that a patient would benefit from surgery or laser around the periorbital region, again, I would not recommend Thermage treatment, as the patient is likely seeking a surgical or resurfacing result. Patients who previously have had a facelift and after 2 to 3 years are beginning to become lax again are usually good candidates for Thermage treatments.

It is important not to promote the procedure as a substitute for surgery, as the procedure can be expensive based on the price of the consumables and the equipment (approximately $70,000 US dollars in Australia). Consumables cost in the range of $200 to $1000 for the tips, and one also must consider the cost of the coolant, the coupling lubricant, the return pad, and temporary marking paper. (*access video on Thermage in the online version of this article at*: http://www.plasticsurgery.theclinics.com/)

CONTRAINDICATIONS TO TREATMENT

Clinically, the only contraindications are for patients who have implanted electronic devices and those taking anti-inflammatory drugs that can impair the collagen remodeling. Other, experience-based contraindications are those related to the patient's expectations as alluded to previously and for those patients who have thin skin, either actinically damaged or with autoimmune disease,

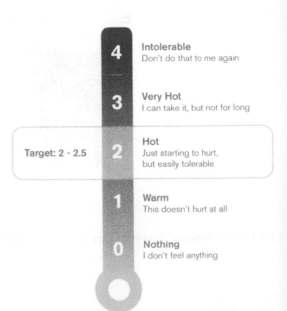

Fig. 5. Patient's verbal response to the heated area where sensitivity controls the dose of radiofrequency delivered. (*Courtesy of* Thermage, Inc., Hayward, CA; with permission.)

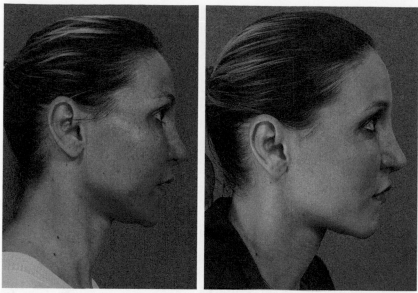

Fig. 6. Before and after Thermage in a 30-year-old neck and jaw line, 2 months after treatment.

or heavy smokers who might incur a compromise in their healing after dermal injury. Many patients have had dermal fillers previously, and it has been shown that it is safe to treat over dermal fillers.[8]

A patient is treated in a dedicated room and is instructed regarding the necessary responses that they should make to the treatment. The patient responds by informing the physician or nurse practitioner what the heat sensations are in the application of the treatment, and this controls the delivery of power from the Thermage machine **(Fig 5)**.

The aim is for the patient to tolerate the treatment as being warm to hot but not one that causes extreme discomfort. By doing this, the patient and the treatment physician or nurse avoid overheating the dermis, causing blistering and at the same time assure therapeutic levels of treatment. Local anesthesia, topical anesthesia, or tumescent infusion are not recommended, nor is intravenous sedation or deep anesthesia, as this removes the patient's ability to inform the nurse or physician of excessive heat sensation. By following these guidelines, I have not had any patient with a blister or contour irregularity after treatment.

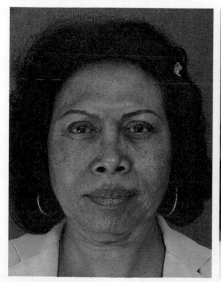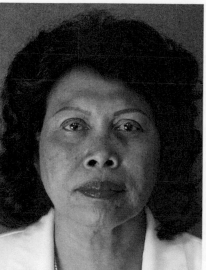

Fig. 7. Before and after Thermage in a 50-year-old neck and jowls, 4 months after treatment.

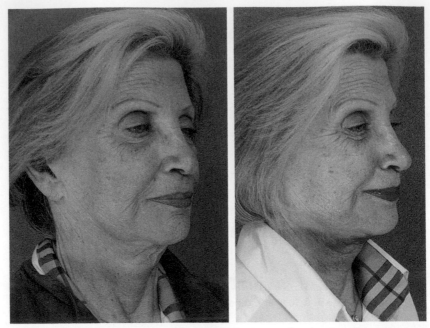

Fig. 8. A 78-year-old woman is shown 3 years after facelift and immediately after Thermage treatment to jowls and neck.

Before beginning the treatment, the patient's individual impedance is automatically measured by the system, and after the grid has been applied, and specific problem areas and desired skin contraction directions marked (vectors), the treatment progresses, noting that in a unified and organized way, some physicians prefer to do one side of the face then the other.

Usually 600 to 800 firings are used in the face and 900 to 1200 in the body. As noted, the grid has circles and squares, and the physician or nurse practitioner uses sequential square circle passes that result in overlapping and more heating. First there is a base pass throughout the whole area, then passes as vectors for elevation of sagging tissues, and then further passes over problem areas such as jowls and submental area, to achieve clinically discernible shrinkage. To promote shrinkage, multiple passes might be given in one area. The treatment should be rapid so as to keep the temperature as high as possible in the treated area.

The usual treatment takes approximately 1 hour. Treatment end points are noted to be slight

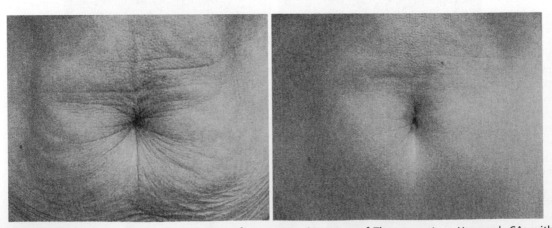

Fig. 9. Thermage of the abdomen, 2 months after surgery. (*Courtesy of* Thermage, Inc., Hayward, CA; with permission.)

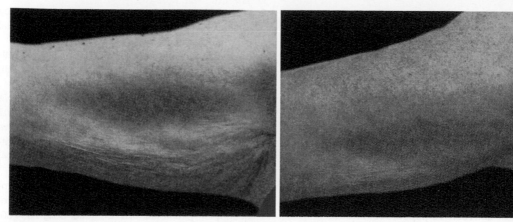

Fig. 10. Thermage of the arms. (*Courtesy of* Thermage, Inc., Hayward, CA; with permission.)

erythema and evidence of firming in the tissues, either the patient putting his or her tongue into the cheek or with a mirror noting the initial tightness that has occurred from the treatment. The procedure is operator-dependent, and the company provides on-site training of operators and certification and then ongoing support for Thermage practitioners.

POST-TREATMENT AFTERCARE

Slight erythema might be treated with 1% hydrocortisone only. Normal skin care regimes can be resumed the following day. Patients are followed up at intervals of 1 and 6 months after their initial treatment. No further treatments are advisable within 6 months. Photographic documentation is important, as results can vary from subtle to dramatic and a studio-like environment with careful digital photography is suggested to be able to document the changes that occur.

After having used the treatment for 3 years, numerous patients have returned after 6 months, as they are impressed with the results and have second treatments.

The skin complexion seems to be improved from the delivery of the radiofrequency to the facial skin, which is another source of patient gratification. Those patients dissatisfied are likely those who were expecting a surgical result and whose practitioners did not determine this before the treatment. Some patients have progressed on to secondary facelift procedures, and there does not seem to be any technical problem performing face-lifting after Thermage treatment to the face.

The main complications noted have been those of contour irregularity with the older machines, particularly over the temporal or cheek regions, where there possibly has been fat atrophy because of the elevated energy levels and single-pass

protocol once used. This is more likely to have occurred in patients who had local anesthetic medication at the time of treatment, which must be discouraged. Blistering is a rare complication.

CLINICAL EXAMPLES

Three cases are shown of Thermage treatment in the face, primarily a young woman, middle-aged woman, and elderly woman after a facelift (**Figs 6–8**).

OTHER AREAS OF THE BODY

The limbs, abdomen, and buttock area have been treated. New, deeper treatment tips have been developed to facilitate more effective treatment in these areas. The results of arm and abdomen are seen, but because less experience is available in these areas by most practitioners, prediction of patient satisfaction is not as reliable as for the face (**Figs. 9** and **10**).

SUMMARY

Radiofrequency tissue tightening by Thermage has become an established technique in the face and eyes for those patients who are optimizing a nonsurgical approach for their surgical rejuvenation. Skin tightening in off-face areas such as arms, thighs, abdomens, and buttocks are also becoming very popular in demand. Over 2300 physicians worldwide are current users of Thermage.

Most likely, these patients are frequent users of fillers or Botox, none of which affect early sagging of the jowls, nasolabial folds, or neck. Here Thermage on a patient who has good-quality skin and early aging, not wishing for an operative procedure, might benefit from and be satisfied by Thermage radiofrequency tissue tightening.

The experience of many plastic surgeons who have integrated this technology into their practice has led to cautious enthusiasm for extending the indications of Thermage to the arms with slight wrinkling, abdomen and periumbilical rhytids, and areas of irregularity in the buttocks, either after liposuction or primarily with cellulite and most recently to body contouring, where the deeper tips might offer modest reshaping in the waist, buttock, hip, and thigh area.

APPENDIX: SUPPLEMENTARY MATERIAL

Supplementary material can be found, in the online version, at doi:10.1016/j.cps.2008.11.006.

REFERENCES

1. Fitzpatrick R, Geronemus R, Goldberg D, et al. Multicenter study of noninvasive radiofrequency for periorbital tissue tightening. Lasers Surg Med 2003;33:232–42.
2. Abraham M, Chiang S, Keller G, et al. Clinical evaluation of non ablative radiofrequency facial rejuvenation. J Cosmet Laser Ther 2004;6:136–44.
3. Fritz M, Counters JT, Zelickson BD. Radiofrequency treatment for middle and lower face laxity. Arch Facial Plast Surg 2004;6:370–3.
4. Koch RJ. Radiofrequency nonablative tissue tightening. Facial Plast Surg Clin North Am 2004;12(3): 339–46.
5. Nahm WK, Su TT, Rotunda A, et al. Objective changes in brow position, superior palpebral crease, peak angle of the eyebrow and jowl surface area after volumetric radiofrequency treatments to half of the face. Dermatol Surg 2004; 30(6):922–8.
6. Ruiz-Esparza J. Noninvasive lower eyelid blepharoplasty—a new technique using nonablative radiofrequency on periorbital skin. Dermatol Surg 2004;30: 125–9.
7. Abraham MT, Mashkevich G. Monopolar radiofrequency skin tightening. Facial Plast Surg Clin North Am 2007;15:169–77.
8. Alan M, Levy R, Pavjoni U, et al. Safety of radiofrequency treatment over human skin previously injected with medium term injectable soft tissue augmentation materials: a controlled pilot trial. Lasers Surg Med 2006;38(3):206–10.

Breast Reconstruction and Augmentation Using Pre-Expansion and Autologous Fat Transplantation

Roger Khouri, MD[a], Daniel Del Vecchio, MD[b],*

KEYWORDS

- Breast reconstruction • Breast augmentation
- Fat grafting • Fat transplantation

The concept of fat grafting for volume enhancement is not a new one. Although surgeons have been injecting fat for years,[1,2] recent focus by clinicians[3] and basic science investigators has generated a groundswell of enthusiasm for a "back to the science" approach to fat transplantation. There is much to study to maximize both graft volume and, more importantly, patient safety. This article outlines the authors' approach to breast deformities using fat grafting, with emphasis on current technique.

FAT GRAFTING: HARVESTING

After Illouz's[4] seminal paper describing the ability to remove fat cells from small port incisions using a cannula, liposuction offered surgeons a low-morbidity new supply of autologous filler. Because many of the variables so important to fat grafting were not well understood at that time, early results were disappointing as it related to volume maintenance.

One of the most frustrating outcomes plastic surgeons experience is often in fat grafting. Despite the same surgeon, the same technique, and the same recipient site, there is a wide variability among volumes maintained over time (**Fig. 1**).

Donor age, donor site, harvesting technique and instrumentation used with harvesting, processing technique, injection technique, and recipient site management both pregrafting and postgrafting

are all vitally important to the success of fat grafting and to maintenance of volume.[5] Looking to the science In the organ transplantation literature may help standardize techniques in this area.

Intuitively, donor (and recipient) age is thought to be a factor in the success of fat grafting. Animal studies in nude mice suggest this to be the case.[6] Data from human fat over a range of donor ages injected subcutaneously into nude immunocompromised mice, suggested higher volume retention in recipients with fat from younger donors. In practice, autologous fat grafting does not afford the opportunity to control for this variable and this may only serve as a prognosticator for patients preoperatively.

Harvesting techniques vary greatly in liposuction and certainly impact cell survival and graft take. Several studies have demonstrated that less suction results in more viable adipocytes.[7] Generally, handheld syringe methods are thought to traumatize adipocytes less and are recommended to harvest fat. In addition, smaller-gauge syringes are recommended so as to avoid fat clumping and to ease in reinjection.

Ostensibly, one might think that surgically resected fat, which is then diced with minimal trauma, maintains cellular integrity better than suctioned fat by any method, and results in better graft take.[8] Ongoing studies are being performed in this area to understand better the role of minimizing graft trauma[9] and there is an opportunity

[a] Dermatology and Plastic Surgery, Key Biscayne, FL, USA
[b] Back Bay Plastic Surgery, 38 Newbury Street, Boston, MA 02116, USA
* Corresponding author.
E-mail address: dandelvecchio@aol.com (D. Del Vecchio).

Clin Plastic Surg 36 (2009) 269–280
doi:10.1016/j.cps.2008.11.009
0094-1298/08/$ – see front matter © 2009 Published by Elsevier Inc

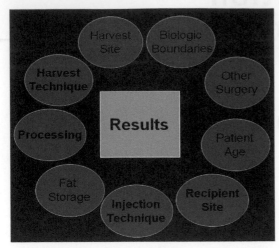

Fig. 1. Fat grafting. Current variables.

to validate this question and potentially to improve instrumentation in this area.

FAT PROCESSING

There have been multiple reports of "percent graft take" by volume.[10] Because of lack of standardization in grafting technique, clinicians must consider rethinking the results of many of these studies. Sixty milliliters of aspirated fat using the tumescent technique decants to a variable aliquot of fat and serum, including blood and crystalloid. Sixty milliliters of aspirate may decant to 30 to 40 mL of fat. When this fat is then centrifuged or rolled on a Telfa pad, two techniques used to concentrate fat further, the resultant fat may reduce to 20 mL by volume. It is not surprising that when fat is grafted, even if all the fat survives, in many cases one has already committed to at best a 30% to 40% volume take, because that is the actual amount of fat that has been inserted by volume.

Although separation by simple decanting uses $1g$ to separate higher-density blood and crystalloid from adipocytes, a high-speed centrifuge uses much higher gravitational forces ($3g$–$5g$) and separates fat from crystalloid extremely well. These centrifuges also require transfer of fat into multiple individual 5- or 10-mL syringes. It has been demonstrated, however, that subjecting adipocytes to $3g$ to $5g$ of centrifugation results in a higher degree of cell death.[11] A compromise between these two techniques that the authors use is manual centrifugation. Prototype devices, similar to the geared concept used in salad spinners, can subject larger volumes of adipocytes to $1g$ to $2g$ forces to separate out unwanted crystalloid better, without subjecting the fat to excessive

($3g$–$5g$ forces) trauma or excessive syringe manipulation (**Fig. 2**).

Subjecting adipocytes to air can potentially damage the cells and can decrease their survival. In addition, the time between harvesting and reinjection increases duration of hypoxia and potentially has an effect on adipocyte survival. Such concerns support the argument that fat grafting in large volumes (unlike those performed for lip or nasolabial folds) might best be accomplished with a team approach. Ostensibly, it is recommended that an assistant or several assistants process fat simultaneously while surgical liposuction harvest is performed.

INJECTION TECHNIQUE

Injection technique also varies and probably plays a role in fat grafting survival. Bolus injections are to be condemned because they defeat the purpose of oxygen diffusion and usually result in fat liquefaction, necrosis, and oil cysts. Dispersing the fat as evenly as possible into as many interstices as possible in the recipient tissue theoretically gives the donor cells the highest chance of maintaining an oxygen diffusion gradient over the critical 3 to 5 days postgrafting.

There are currently several preferred techniques of grafting fat into the breast. The authors' preferred technique, the "mapping" technique, involves the use of small (3-mL) syringes handheld and connected directly to a 16-gauge blunt needle. Markings are made in the recipient areas (**Fig. 3**) to aid in a systematic injection. An exact amount of fat (1–2 mL) is then injected slowly on withdrawal. The needle is then inserted into another adjacent tunnel and the process is repeated. This technique is more deliberate and exact but does take more time. In addition, it requires the operator to deploy the plunger and withdraw the needle at the same time.

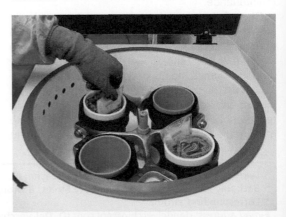

Fig. 2. Manual centrifugation in closed IV collection bag system.

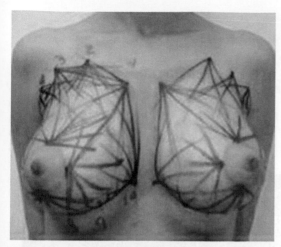

Fig. 3. Mapping technique of fat injection.

A second technique is the "reverse liposuction" method. A 30-mL syringe containing prepared fat is connected to short intravenous extension tubing and is connected to an injection needle. An assistant depresses the plunger at a desired rate (as directed by the surgeon) while the surgeon focuses only on the motion and location of the needle. In this manner, a large volume of fat can be randomly dispersed into the recipient site in a shorter period of time. It is vitally important to keep the needle under motion at all times and to keep the injection speed low to avoid bolus injections. When starting out with fat grafting to the breast the mapping technique is generally advised. To date there are no data suggesting one technique is superior.

Because many reports suggest at best 30% fat take, one controversy in fat grafting has been whether or not to overcorrect. Overcorrection historically seemed alluring because one might reach a desired end point knowing a significant amount of adipocytes would not survive. It is believed, however, that the increased interstitial pressure created in most cases results in lack of oxygen diffusion and cell death, potentially of all the cells.

Indeed, some of the best clinical results in fat grafting have been demonstrated by those who promote small serial volume sessions of fat grafting. The evidence suggests that this approach is successful because it respects the interstitial pressure limitations of the recipient site and in doing so, promotes diffusion during the initial critical days postgrafting.

THE ROLE OF THE RECIPIENT SITE

Recipient site management has only recently been suggested as a potential important variable in fat grafting. From the general surgery trauma literature and from hand and upper extremity trauma, the importance of compartment pressure and grave consequences of interstitial pressure are well understood. If it is possible to increase the volume of the interstitial space before fat grafting, it is potentially feasible to inject a larger volume of graft into the recipient site before reaching high interstitial pressures.

Experience with the vacuum-assisted closure as a means of wound management has proved that microangiogenesis is a direct result of negative mechanical pressure.[12] The extensive vacuum-assisted closure data on vascular in-growth coupled with the MRI findings from BRAVA-expanded breasts support the authors' thesis that increased microcirculation, combined with the larger interstitial space created by the expansion, may both contribute to the potential for increased fat volumes and increased diffusion gradients. Although such postulates are currently being considered for animal study, mechanical difficulties related to immobilization of vacuum domes on animal subjects remain a significant challenge (**Fig. 4**).

The BRAVA bra was initially developed in the 1990s to generate a nonsurgical negative pressure breast enhancement. The device generates a negative pressure that creates an inflow of fluid, in this case interstitial fluid, and increased vascularity. The device was typically worn nightly under a low negative pressure, and over 4 to 6 weeks breast enlargement of a cup size on average was achieved. Once the device was discontinued from use, however, breast size regressed to the pre-expansion baseline.

When used as a recipient site modulator before fat grafting, pre-expansion is thought to generate a more supple skin envelope, especially in reconstruction cases and in cases of irradiated tissue. In addition, the increased interstitial space is believed to allow for a larger volume of fat to be grafted while still dispersing the cells with oxygen-rich recipient site tissue. Clinically, the authors aim for a twofold to threefold increase in volume before grafting (**Fig. 5**).

Postoperatively, skin grafts are immobilized to promote secure apposition of the donor cells to the recipient wound bed. This promotes an adequate diffusion gradient and greater likelihood that angiogenesis occurs. Searing of the graft or movement of any type in this initial 3 to 5 days can prove fatal for a skin graft. It is believed that immobilization of the transplanted adipocyte can best be accomplished with mild external negative pressure. The authors are currently advocating use of the BRAVA bra for 5 to 7 days postgrafting.

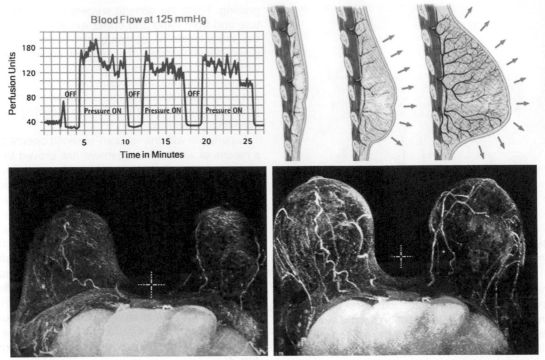

Fig. 4. VAC data demonstrate increased circulatory flow with negative pressure (*top left*). (*Data from* KCI.) The theoretical effect of negative pressure on breast circulation (*top right*). MRI of breasts pre-expansion (*bottom left*). Postexpansion using BRAVA (*bottom right*). Note the real increase in vessel caliber and number postexpansion.

Not only does the mild negative pressure serve to immobilize the fat in its interstitial space, it also may help with angiogenesis as has been demonstrated with the vacuum-assisted closure. Lastly, the domes of the external expander BRAVA unit help protect the newly grafted tissue from external movement and trauma.

IMPROVED INSTRUMENTATION

In 1980, when Illouz first described the liposuction technique, 10-mm cannulae were described. Thirty years later, clinicians are now rapidly removing fat using 12-gauge cannulae with multiple side ports, in a less traumatic manner (**Fig. 6**).

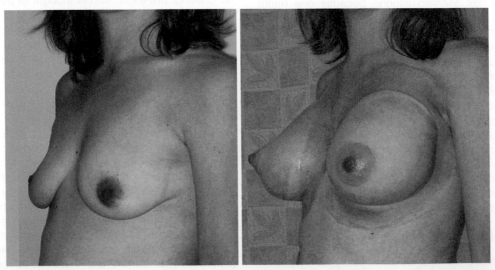

Fig. 5. A threefold to fourfold volume expansion of the recipient site is possible and desirable before fat grafting.

Fig. 6. Commonly used 12-gauge cannula for fat harvesting.

CELL PRESERVATION TECHNIQUES FROM TRANSPLANTATION LITERATURE

In the solid organ transplantation, cell preservation is maximized by hypothermia and extracorporeal perfusion during organ transfer using a variety of solutions. One such solution, University of Wisconsin Solution,[13] is a highly concentrated potassium solution that reduces cellular metabolism in the solid organ during its period of cellular hypoxia and anoxia, and is thought to reduce cellular death following reperfusion in the recipient site. This highly concentrated potassium solution is not used in vivo, but is used to perfuse the solid organ while in transit and in preparation for transplantation. In general surgery shock and trauma, a variety of solutions are known to improve reperfusion and improve cell survival following resuscitation. These represent just a few starting points for several potential strategies that are suitable for study for possible adoption in maximizing techniques of fat transplantation. Current research is underway to identify optimal solutions in this area.[14]

BREAST RECONSTRUCTION AND AUGMENTATION: THE EMERGING ROLE OF THE RECIPIENT SITE AND FAT GRAFTING
The State of Mastectomy Surgery in the United States

Annually in the United States, there are approximately 182,000 newly diagnosed cases of breast cancer that require some type of surgical procedure to treat breast cancer.[15] These generally represent some form of mastectomy or lumpectomy; however, there are approximately 57,000 breast reconstructions performed a year in the United States.[16] If one assumes that all these reconstructions are performed for immediate (or in the same year of the mastectomy) reconstruction, at best only 31% of patients are receiving some form of breast reconstruction. This number is probably lower because many of the reconstructions are performed on cases diagnosed and surgically treated in prior years. This also means that every decade, approximately 1.2 million women are electing to do nothing about their postsurgical breast deformity. Why do such a high percentage of breast cancer surgery patients elect to do nothing following lumpectomy or mastectomy? One postulate is that the degree of morbidity of the reconstruction outweighs the

perceived aesthetic improvement over the existing deformity.

In this orphaned population, a low-morbidity procedure to reconstruct breast defects that results in significant aesthetic improvement represents a large opportunity.

The State of Breast Augmentation Surgery in the United States

An adequate discussion of augmentation with breast implants is beyond the context of this article. It is interesting to consider, however, the risk-reward analysis similar to that outlined in the patient after breast cancer surgery.

Reviewing available statistics, there were approximately 348,500 cosmetic breast augmentations performed in the United States in 2007. In addition, retail data from *Consumer Reports* suggests that at least 34% of women in the United States own padded bras.[17] Based on standard assumptions about the United States population and the percent of women of adult age, for every women who undergoes a cosmetic breast enhancement, there are over 100 women who, for whatever reason, would like their breasts to appear larger in some way. The same rational for nonsurgery (padded bras) may also exist as it does for breast reconstruction. Besides financial issues, concerns over artificial implants, and other personal concerns, a remaining variable is that the degree of morbidity of the augmentation does not outweigh the aesthetic improvement over the existing aesthetic concern. As in the case of reconstruction, a low-morbidity procedure to augment breasts that results in significant improvement represents a large number of potential patients, much larger than the reconstruction population.

Patient Evaluation: Medical

The patient presenting for breast reconstruction or augmentation with autologous fat grafting should be evaluated for associated medical conditions that might otherwise exclude them from safely undergoing a liposuction procedure. Acutely, the liposuction aspect of the intervention is probably higher in morbidity than that of the breast fat grafting. Smokers are generally not advised as candidates for breast reconstruction with fat grafting with pre-expansion. Donor site fat is evaluated for the likely availability of fully processed fat.

Irradiated patients have been successfully treated using BRAVA pre-expansion. In irradiated reconstructions, the skin envelope expands more slowly and serial expansion and injection sessions are required. It is generally advised to begin breast reconstruction in nonirradiated mastectomy patients and first become familiar with these techniques before embarking on treating irradiated defects. The assessment of the opposite breast is addressed with the same principles as for any breast reconstruction.

Patient Evaluation: The Role of Compliance

Animal studies with negative pressure pre-expansion are challenging because of difficulties maintaining a device in animal subjects. The same can be said for patients with regards to BRAVA pre-expansion. There is no substitute for sustained moderate to high negative pressure pre-expansion to maximize pre–fat grafting volume of the recipient site. Indeed, the earliest versions of the negative pressure pumps were low-voltage battery-operated devices that exerted a low negative pressure. These patients exhibited less dramatic pregrafting expansion when compared with more powerful pumps currently used. These pumps are similar in negative pressure and in terms of size and portability as the vacuum-assisted closure pump, and have demonstrated a dose response curve with regards to both pre-expansion volume and to overall fat volume results postgrafting.

Based on experience with the dose response data, the authors believe there is no substitute for adequate pre-expansion. The degree and extent of pregrafting expansion is directly proportional to the amount of grafting possible to maintain a physiologic interstitial pressure. Last minute "cramming" on part of the patient has been experienced and does not result in successful preparation. It is ultimately the responsibility of the surgeon adequately to select, educate, coach, and troubleshoot their patients to ensure adequate and optimal pre-expansion. Patients should spend as much time in-office the first time they use their bras to ensure they are properly educated and motivated to use the device.

BASELINE VOLUME CONSIDERATIONS

The more breast and subcutaneous tissue there is to begin with, the easier it is to volume expand with negative pressure. In addition, the less scar damaged (nonirradiated) the tissue is, the easier it is to expand with negative pressure. The following cases serve as extreme examples (**Box 1**).

Box 1
Examples of baseline volume considerations

Case A: Augmentation

Existing breasts, 250 mL size. Desired final breast volume, 500 mL. Plan: pre-expansion to desired volume, then graft. Percent expansion = (500–250)/250 = 100%.

Case B: Reconstruction

Existing breast skin, subcutaneous fat 50 mL size. Desired volume, 500 mL. Plan: pre-expansion to desired volume, then graft. Percent expansion = (500–50)/50 = 900%.

The number of sessions for Case A may be one, whereas the number may be four to five for Case B.

Preferred Techniques

BRAVA: recipient site preparation

In cases of mastectomy and for augmentation, the BRAVA dome is placed for 3 to 4 weeks and is worn 12 hours daily. For the last 4 to 5 days before fat grafting, it is advised to wear the domes 24 hours a day. Circumferential pressure at the edges of the domes can create skin sensitivity and this should be explained to patients who should reduce the degree of negative pressure. Nonirradiated skin and subcutaneous tissue has greater potential for parenchymal expansion than cases performed in irradiated tissue, which requires more serial sessions (**Fig. 7**).

The location and degree of body fat available is analyzed to evaluate the existence of an adequate amount of donor fat. Because there are so many variables (amount of tumescence, degree of bleeding, time allowed for tumescent solution to set) it is impossible to formulate a standard ratio of aspirate to actual processed fat by volume. As a conservative rule, four to five times the desired volume of fat needed for grafting should be available to be harvested as aspirate. For example, if reconstruction using 400 mL of fat is planned, the patient should be able to render at least 1600 to 2000 mL of aspirate to ensure adequate donor material.

$$Aspirate = 5 \times Graft;\ 2000\ mL = 5 \times 400\ mL$$

Considering the pre-expansion effort the patient must tolerate, it is always better to have more than less fat available.

In the case of augmentation with 300 mL of fat on each side, a minimum of 3000 mL of aspirate is recommended. Patients with body mass indexes as low as 23 to 24 have been successfully

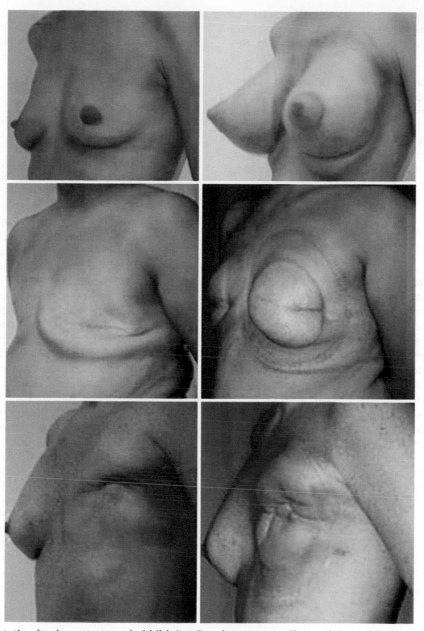

Fig. 7. Augmentation (*top*), mastectomy (*middle*), irradiated mastectomy (*bottom*) sites with pre-expansion. After 3 to 4 weeks, note the varying range of expansion possible in each category.

treated. The lower the body mass index, the greater the number of donor sites (abdomen, knees, thighs, and so forth) that must be entered to harvest adequate amounts of aspirate and fat.

Lipografting: preoperative planning
On the day of surgery patients are photographed and marked as usual for liposuction. Markings are made for injection sites on the breasts and lines are made on the breast mound to ensure proper dispersion of the fat grafts. Patients are

brought into the operating room still wearing the BRAVA bra to maximize expansion closer to the point of injection. Once all the fat is harvested and processed, the Bra is removed, the site is prepared and redraped, and injection takes place.

Harvesting and collection
Fat is harvested using a 12-gauge blunt cannula with multiple side ports. Syringe aspiration is used as opposed to high negative pressure machine techniques. To avoid desiccation,

a closed system is used, transferring the fat from the syringe directly into an empty sterile intravenous bag by an extension tubing setup (**Fig. 8**).

Processing

Once an adequate amount of aspirate is harvested, the collected intravenous bags are decanted of unwanted fluid and are placed into a manual centrifuge. This manual centrifuge further separates fluid from the adipocytes without subjecting the cells to excessive handling, desiccation, or trauma, as is postulated with high-speed centrifugation in small syringes.

Once the fat is properly processed in this manner, the fat is then drawn back into 3- or 5-mL syringes from the intravenous collection bags using a three-way stopcock, and grafting begins.

Recipient site techniques: needle band release

Multiple radial needle insertions are made around the breast mound to disperse the grafted adipocytes maximally and to ensure as many different planes as possible. Before grafting the fat, if there are breast shaping issues that need to be addressed these can be performed at this time.

In many breasts, fibrous ligamentous tissue or bands distort the breast mound, such as in constricted inframammary folds or in the case of tubular breast deformities. Because expansion of the parenchymal space places these bands under high tension, it facilitates the transaction of these bands using an 18-gauge needle, simply by inserting the needle in the area of the band and through proprioception, "feeling" the blade of the needle cut the band. In this manner, it is possible to "expand" or "release" these constrictions further internally in a manner similar to the external release of a burn scar contracture. The inframammary fold can be lowered in constricted inframammary folds, and the constricted bases of tubular breasts can be widened in this manner. It is important not to overrelease these bands, because too large a dead space might ensue. This reduces the interstices of the tissue and reduces the surface-to-volume characteristics of the recipient site.

Injection technique

Bolus injections are to be condemned because they defeat the purpose of oxygen diffusion and usually result in fat liquefaction and necrosis.

The mapping technique previously described involves the use of small (3-mL) syringes handheld and connected directly to a 16-gauge blunt needle. Through the multiple radial needle insertions around the breast mound, the needle is advanced in the subcutaneous plane and an exact amount of fat (1–2 mL) is then injected slowly on withdrawal. The needle is then inserted into another adjacent tunnel and the process is repeated.

Injection into the prepectoral fat and the subcutaneous fat is performed in as many different depth planes as the recipient tissue tolerates. In the case of mastectomy, the first session of grafting allows fewer planes of grafting and reasonable volumes during the first session (150–250 mL) should be planned. For subsequent sessions, there are more potential planes, because a thicker interstitial space exists. Generally, the more parenchyma one has to begin with, the larger volumes of fat that can be grafted. For first session reconstruction after mastectomy, 150 to 250 mL of fat can be expected. For augmentation or in subsequent grafting sessions in reconstruction, 200 to 300 mL can be planed. For irradiated cases, one should be extremely careful not to overgraft and should expect a minimum of four to five sessions.

In no cases (breast augmentation, treating a lumpectomy defect, breast asymmetry, or any other cases where any breast tissue remains) is it ever recommended to inject fat directly into breast tissue.

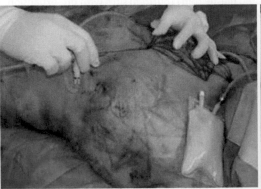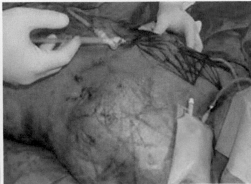

Fig. 8. Closed system method of collection and fat replantation.

POSTOPERATIVE MANAGEMENT

Patients are instructed to wear the BRAVA bra 5 to 7 days postgrafting. This potentially helps with graft immobilization, potentiates neovascularization, and definitely protects the breast from external pressure or trauma.

REPRESENTATIVE RESULTS
Breast Reconstruction

The patient in **Fig. 9** had bilateral mastectomy (radical on the right) and had four serial sessions of BRAVA pre-expansion and fat grafting sessions of 150 mL each time.

Breast Reconstruction for Severe Asymmetry

The 20-year-old patient in **Fig. 10** had a giant congenital nevus excised as a child and demonstrated hypomastia on the left, documented by MRI. She underwent 3 weeks of BRAVA pre-expansions to increase her parenchymal space and to increase the vertical skin envelope deficiency. She underwent a single session with grafting of 300 mL into the left breast. Her postoperative result at 6 months reveals retention of grafted fat volume.

Breast Augmentation: Postpartum Deflation

The 33-year-old patient shown in **Fig. 11** desired larger breasts after having several children and experiencing some mild deflation. Although she wore a padded bra and desired a cup size increase in volume, she did not wish to have breast augmentation with implants. She underwent 3 weeks of BRAVA pre-expansions to increase her parenchymal space bilaterally. She underwent a single session with grafting of 250 mL into

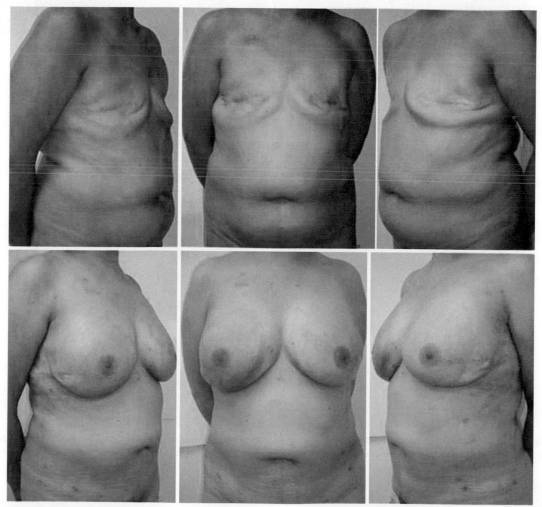

Fig. 9. Patient with bilateral mastectomy and BRAVA pre-expansion reconstruction; three sessions, 600 mL total.

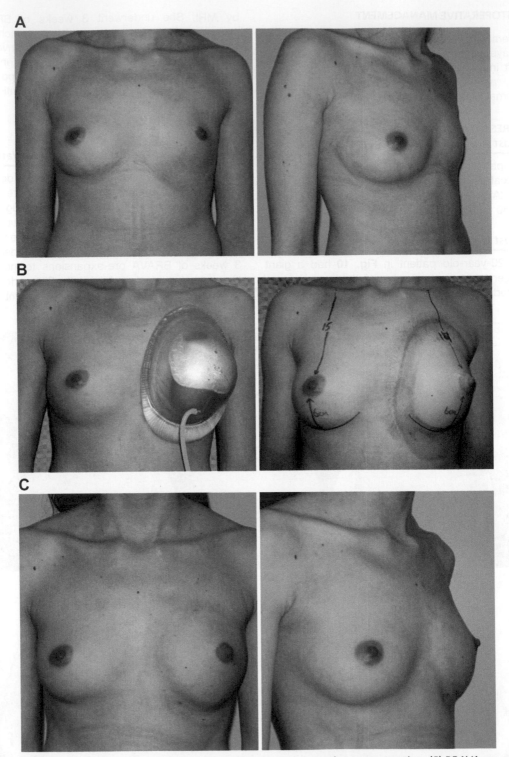

Fig. 10. (*A*) Patient with severe breast asymmetry and BRAVA pre-expansion reconstruction. (*B*) BRAVA pre-expansion increases parenchyma and skin envelope. (*C*) Six months after 280 mL of fat transplanted into the left breast.

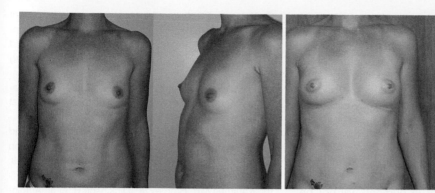

Fig. 11. The patient is shown pre-expansion (*left*) and 9 months after fat grafting (*right*).

each breast. At 9 months postgrafting, she demonstrates adequate volume maintenance.

A COMPARISON OF BREAST RECONSTRUCTION USING THREE TECHNIQUES

Table 1 helps delineate some of the main differences between currently popular reconstruction options and breast reconstruction using pre-expansion and autologous fat transplantation.

CONTROVERSIAL TOPICS

At the time of this communication, it is early days in breast augmentation and reconstruction using fat transplantation. There are more questions than there are answers, and it is easier to ask than to answer the questions. The following represent some of the biggest controversies and challenges facing this technique in the near, medium, and long term.

Imaging and Detection of Breast Cancer

In 1987, the American Society of Plastic Surgeons position paper strongly condemned fat grafting to the breast suggesting fat grafting would distort the ability of breast cancer detection. Breast fat grafting has been demonstrated to sometimes result in microcalcifications.[18] Although many of these calcifications are believed to be distinguishable from calcifications of higher grade that are suggestive of malignancy, unnecessary biopsies have resulted from this effect.

Risk of Cancer: The Aromatase Question

It is well known that one in nine women experience breast cancer in their lifetime. Although it takes a nearly impossible study size to prove causality or statistical significance, the question has been raised that aromatase, a breakdown product of adipocyte necrosis, might cause breast cancer. The validity of this is unknown.

Table 1
Differences among breast reconstruction options

	Tissue Expander/Implant	TRAM	BRAVA
Pain level	Moderate	High	Low
No. procedures	2	1–2	1–4
General anesthesia	2	1–2	0–1
Office visits for expansion	3–5	None	None
Expansion type	Serial, office based	None	Continuous
Recipient site skin	Thinned	NA	Thickened
Hospital days	0–1	3–5	None
Donor site morbidity	NA	High	Liposuction, bonus
Patient compliance	Patient passive	Passive	Compliance is key
Reoperation tolerance	Moderately possible	Unlikely	Simple
Cost to system	Moderate	High	Low

What is known is that surgeons have performed thousands of procedures over the past 20 years in large numbers that cause fat cell necrosis. Despite thousands of TRAM flaps, with a high degree of fat necrosis in zone II and III, breast liposuctions, and breast reductions, there is no evidence, retrospective or prospective, that these procedures are associated with a higher degree of breast cancer.

Such facts should not be sufficient, however, as to ignore the question of safety. Although there are currently models being developed to evaluate this carcinogenic potential in an animal model, the reality is that the answer in humans will not be available before the widespread use of this technique. Any patients entertaining any breast fat grafting, including reconstruction patients and breast augmentation patients, must be given full informed consent as to the unknown risks of the technique. Although many suggest this technique not be performed without the approval of an internal review board, the reality is that the technique is already being performed.

There is an unmet clinical need for more institutional review board–approved, multisite studies that can demonstrate reproducible and safe results by many independent surgeons. Such collective data in the literature will eventually help delineate the safety issues as they relate to carcinogenesis and cancer detection.

REFERENCES

1. Czerny V [Plastischer ersatz der brustdruse durch ein lipom]. Zentralbl Chir 1895;27:72.
2. Hinderer UT, Del Rio JL. Erich Lexer's mammaplasty. Aesthetic Plast Surg 1992;16:101.
3. Coleman SR, Saboeiro AP. Fat grafting to the breast revisited: safety and efficacy. Plast Reconstr Surg 2007;119(3):775–85.
4. Illouz YG. Body contouring by lipolysis: a five year experience with over 3000 cases. Plast Reconstr Surg 1983;72(5):591–7.
5. Shiffman MA, Mirrafati S. Fat transfer techniques: the effect of harvest and transfer methods on adipocyte viability and review of the literature. Dermatol Surg 2001;27:819–26.
6. Bucky LP, Godek CP. Discussion of "Behavior of fat grafts and recipient areas with enhanced vascularity: an experimental study" by Baran CN, et al. Plast Reconstr Surgery 2002;109(5):1652.
7. Kononas TC, Bucky LP, Hurley C, et al. The fate of suctioned and surgically removed fat after reimplantation for soft-tissue augmentation: a volumetric and histologic study in the rabbit. Plast Reconstr Surg 1993;91(5):763–8.
8. Guyuron B, Majzoub Ramsey K. Facial augmentation with core fat graft: a preliminary report. Plast Reconstr Surg 2007;120(1):295–302.
9. Billings E Jr, May JW Jr. Historical review and present status of free fat graft autotransplantation in Plast Reconstr Surg. Plast Reconstr Surg 1989; 83(2):368–81.
10. Kaufman MR, Bradley JP, Dickinson B, et al. Autologous fat transfer national consensus survey: trends in techniques for harvest, preparation, and application, and perception of short- and long-term results. Plast Reconstr Surg 2007;119(1):323–31.
11. Kurita M, Matsumoto D, Shigeura T, et al. Influences of centrifugation on cells and tissues in liposuction aspirates: optimized centrifugation for lipotransfer and cell isolation. Plast Reconstr Surg 2008;121(3): 1033–41.
12. Morykwas MJ, Argenta LC, Shelton-Brown EI, et al. Vacuum assisted closure: a new method for wound control and treatment: animal studies and basic foundation. Ann Plast Surg 1997;38(6): 553–62.
13. Agarwal A, Goggins M, Pescovitz M, et al. Comparison of histidine-tryptophan ketoglutarate and University of Wisconsin solutions as primary preservation in renal allografts undergoing pulsatile perfusion. Transplant Proc 2005;37(5):2016–9.
14. Murphy AD, McCormack MC, Bichara D. Poloxamer 188 significantly decreases muscle necrosis in a murine hindlimb model of ischemia reperfusion injury. Presented at Northeastern Society of Plastic Surgeons, Philadelphia, Oct 3, 2008.
15. National Breast Cancer Organization. Available at: www.yme.org/information/breast_cancer_news/breast_cancer_statistics.php.
16. American Society of Plastic Surgeons. Available at: www.plasticsurgery.org/media/statistics/loader.cfm?url=/commonspot/security/getfile.cfm&;PageID=29287.
17. Available at: coupdefoudrelingerie.blogspot.com/2008/05/new-bra-statistics-from-consumer.html.
18. Uchiyama N, Miyagawa K, Matsue H, et al. The radiographic findings of the breast after augmentation by fat injection. Japanese Journal of Clinical Radiology 2000;45(5):675–9.

APTOS Suture Lifting Methods: 10 Years of Experience

Marlen Sulamanidze, MD[a,b], Georgii Sulamanidze, MD[b,*]

KEYWORDS

- Aptos thread method • Aptos needle method
- Aptos spring method

The process of facial aging is manifested as uneven ptosis of the skin and subcutaneous tissues located above and lateral to the nasolabial fold and the superciliary, buccal, mental, and submental areas.

For various reasons, gravitational sagging of soft tissue occurs, with the resulting appearance of overhanging eyebrows, lachrymal grooves, deepening nasolabial folds, and the beginning of marionette lines, followed by aggravation and ptosis of the angle of the mouth and mental areas becoming more pronounced ("hanging lips").

For a long time these deformities were corrected only by radical interventions: cutaneous, superficial musculoaponeurotic system (SMAS), and periosteal and subperiosteal face lift.[1–4]

In any face lift technique, the medial portions of the face uncrumple incompletely. **Fig. 1** shows that to the edge of the mobilized skin–cutaneous flap a mechanical force is applied and it is extended to the maximum, with each of the marked, initially 3-cm long portions having elongated to a different degree. The farther the portion is away from the point of force application, the less it extends.

Understanding the cause of this factor, we decided to develop a method of tissue extension in which the flap extends evenly along the whole length. Knowledge of the topographic anatomy and clinical experience persuaded us that on separate portions of the face the layers of soft tissues could be easily moved with no mobilization thereof, with the skin capable of shrinking under certain conditions.

Barbed threads have long been used in medicine to suture tendons and close wound edges; however, operations on lifting facial tissues by means of such threads to rejuvenate were first proposed by us as long ago as 1998 (**Fig. 2**). The name Aptos (anti- ptosis), as we called these threads, was then given to all products and technologies of minimally invasive lifting, which were developed and implemented in practice.[5,6]

MATERIALS AND METHODS

Aptos Thread, Aptos Thread 2G, Aptos Needle, Aptos Needle 2G, Aptos Spring: manufactured by the CHIRAMAX Ltd. (Czech Republic), the product possessing a European Certificate.

The needle—a guide of the spinal needle type measuring 1.1 × 100 mm, manufactured by the TSK–Supra SIMS Portex Ltd.

Patients: a total of 4580 people; of these, 4388 women and 192 men operated on in our clinic by the same surgical team between January 1988 and December 2007. The patients' ages varied from 31 to 77 years. The age- and sex-related distribution is shown in **Table 1**.

Financial Disclosure: Dr. Marlen Sulamanidze and Dr. Georgii Sulamanidze are the Chiefs of APTOS.
[a] Department of Plastic and Reconstructive Surgery, Central Hospital No. 165, 3rd Administration of the Russian Federation Health Ministry, Tbilisi, Georgia
[b] Limited Liability Company APTOS, V. Orbeliani str 18, 0105, Tbilisi, Georgia
* Corresponding author. V. Orbeliani str 18, 0105, Tbilisi, Georgia.
E-mail address: gracia@aptos.ru (G. Sulamanidze).

Clin Plastic Surg 36 (2009) 281–306
doi:10.1016/j.cps.2008.12.003
0094-1298/08/$ – see front matter © 2009 Elsevier Inc. All rights reserved.

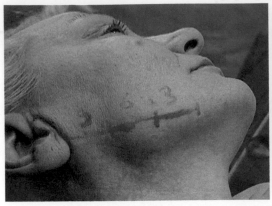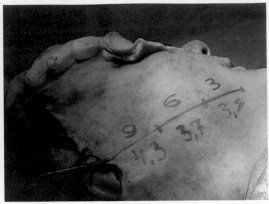

Fig. 1. Experiment that shows different expansions of mobilized cellulocutaneous layer areas through application of mechanical force.

Aptos Thread Method

We performed the first experiments using threads that were provided with barbs directed unilaterally and fixed to a long needle. Through a small incision in the temporal area, we pulled several threads subcutaneously. After the lower thread and needle emerged to the surface of the skin, the remainder of each lower thread was cut off, and, after moderate pulling, the upper thread was sutured to the fascia of the temporal muscle. The same technique was used to pull the soft

tissues of the submaxillary and cervical regions with fixation of the upper end of the thread to the periosteum of the mastoid process (**Fig. 3**).

Later in 1998, we improved this technique slightly by devising a needleless thread with converging barbs, which was introduced under the skin by means of a guiding needle, which made it possible to abandon incisions (**Fig. 4**). Such a thread introduced subcutaneously is fixed in soft tissues because of the barbs converging toward the middle thereof, carrying subcutaneous fat, pulling it together and distributing it evenly

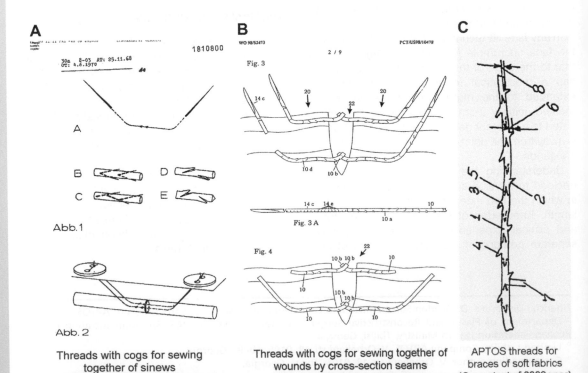

A

Abb. 1

Threads with cogs for sewing together of sinews
(The German patent of 1968 year)

Abb. 2

B

Fig. 3

Fig. 3 A

Fig. 4

Threads with cogs for sewing together of wounds by cross-section seams
(The American May, 1997 year)

C

APTOS threads for braces of soft fabrics
(Our patent of 2002 year)

Fig. 2. (A–C) Diagrams from patents.

Table 1
Age- and sex-related distribution of patients who underwent Aptos suture lifts between January 1988 and December 2007

| Gender | Number (%) of Patients in Each Age Group | | | | |
	31–40 years old	41–50 years old	51–60 years old	≥61	Total
Female	115 (26.1)	167 (37.9)	114 (25.9)	44 (10)	440
Male	3 (7.7)	29 (74.35)	7 (17.9)	0	39
Total	118 (26.5)	196 (40.9)	121 (25.2)	44 (9.2)	479

along the whole length, thus creating the effect of lifting or obtaining a high contour of soft tissues.

Initially, we used this technique on virtually all portions of the face and neck. During long-term practice, however, we concluded that the appropriate use of this method was only for creation of a high contour of the midface soft tissues and lifting of the mental area. Accordingly, we developed an optimal marking of the skin, taking into consideration anatomic and functional peculiarities of the portion concerned and the pathogenesis of the deformity involved (**Fig. 5**).

We managed to obtain better outcomes in 35- to 50-year-old patients who had clear, not very thick skin, with no pronounced atrophy of subcutaneous fat and moderate manifestations of soft tissue ptosis (no sharply pronounced nasolabial folds, overhanging of soft tissue bolsters above them, mild distortions of the suborbital contours in the form of lachrymal grooves, and the presence of hanging lips), who for various reasons refused classic face lift operations. Mainly, these were the patients who wished mild lifting barely visible to other people. These were also patients who had previously undergone cutaneous rhytidoplasty and were not satisfied with the outcome obtained because the facial lifting had been poorly pronounced in the midface portions and high volume of the buccozygomatic regions was not attained.

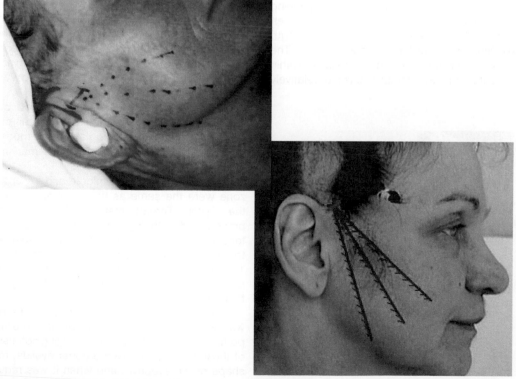

Fig. 3. Our first experiment in Aptos lifting.

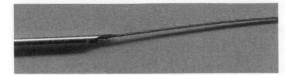

Fig. 4. Aptos thread and guide needle.

Surgical Procedure

To lift the mental regions, the threads were implanted parallel to the mandibular edge with slight arch-like sagging within the area of the hanging lip. Doing so, we simultaneously solved the problem of lifting and redistribution of the skin and subcutaneous fat of the hanging lips. The depth of the thread's implantation varied depending on the thickness of the skin, fat, and the degree of involutional alterations, but obligatorily within fatty tissue, which is thicker closer to the skin.

The main task we accomplished while lifting the midface area was to create a new high contour of the buccozygomatic region by elevation of the ptosed soft tissues situated between the nasolabial fold and lachrymal groove. Movement of the cheek upward and slightly laterally obtained a more smoothed-out nasolabial fold and lachrymal groove.

This effect was achieved by placing the threads within subcutaneous fat in the form of comparatively steep arches followed by straightening them by pulling the ends and accordingly even closing together of soft tissues along the length of the threads toward the middle thereof. The effect was even more enhanced because within the middle part the threads passed relatively

deep, catching SMAS and together with it elevated fatty tissues from the depth toward the surface.

While gaining experience, we planned ways of further developing thread-mediated lifting, with the goals of simplifying the operational technique, enhancing the power of lifting, achieving long-standing results that would persist over time, and decreasing the risk for complications and undesirable effects.

Aptos Thread 2G Method

In 2002, we again returned to the idea of using a single product (ie, a needle with a thread); however, the new suture material was distinguished by the presence of two needles to the ends of which were attached one thread provided with converging barbs—Aptos Thread 2G (**Fig. 6**A). This appliance made it possible to increase the thread's arm of force twofold, and thus to obtain the power and stability of the lifting. An important novelty herein was that these threads were coupled by temporary soldering so that in this position their pointed tips constituted a single whole (**Fig. 6**B). Implementation of the idea of the coupled needles and a novel technique of the operation made it possible to place the threads with no cutaneous incisions through a puncture, obtaining no skin in-drawings in the place of the thread's bend: both needles were stuck into the skin with the common tip, to be detached under the skin at the required depth and only thereafter advanced in the opposite directions. (*access video on Aptos Thread 2G for the eyebrow in the online version of this article at:* http://www.plasticsurgery.theclinics.com/)

The Aptos Thread 2G method yielded better results during operations of lifting the tail of the eyebrow and mental sagging and more moderate results in the midface area. Optimal marking of the skin is shown in (**Fig. 7**).

The indications for the middle and lower facial zone were the same as those for application of the Aptos Thread method, but with more pronounced pathology. In the midface zone, we tended not so much to create a high volume as to distribute soft tissues upward and laterally. The Aptos Thread 2G was also applied when the patient wished a more radical and lasting lifting than the Aptos Thread.

In the area of the eyebrow, Aptos Thread 2G was used in cases of moderate ptosis of the lateral portions of the eyebrows, overhanging soft tissues of these portions above the upper eyelids, round shape of the eyebrow, and when it was required to remove signs of "watering" eyes.

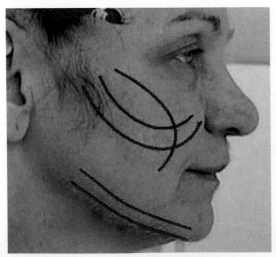

Fig. 5. Method for marking of Aptos thread.

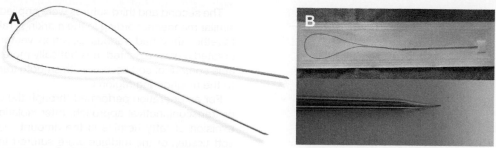

Fig. 6. (*A*) Diagram of Aptos Thread 2G. (*B*) Aptos Thread 2G.

Surgical Procedure

To lift the lateral portion of the eyebrow, the coupled needles were inserted into the skin of the temporal region to the fascia of the temporal muscle, to be detached herein and pulled apart. One of them was advanced to a greater depth to catch the fascia and returned back to the subcutaneous space. Then the threaded needles were alternately advanced along the marked contour to emerge in the marked points, evenly pulling the thread from the both sides, achieving the required shape of the eyebrow, with certain hypercorrection. Doing so, the bend of the thread in the place of entry of the coupled needles was submerged under the skin, tightly holding onto the temporal muscle fascia.

The 2G threads were implanted in the midface and mental regions according to the presented marking and the same guidelines that were described in the section concerning the operative procedure according to the Aptos Thread method. The differences concern the moment of insertion

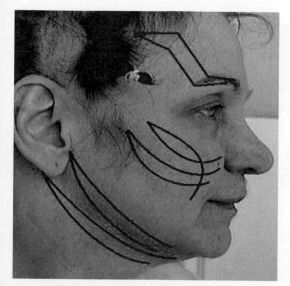

Fig. 7. Marking of Aptos Thread 2G.

of the needles under the skin: it is important to insert the needles into subcutaneous fat in the area of the zygomatic arch, to separate them there and to pull them apart so as to encompass the fascial bands (reference points) with the place of bending of the thread and only thereafter alternately pass the threaded needles according to the marking. The same guidelines are given while lifting the mental area, only the bend of the thread should catch on the fascia of the parotid salivary gland.

Aptos Needle Method

While gaining experience, we noted that some rejuvenating and lifting operations required suturing through soft tissues in the form of a loop or purse (ie, return of the thread back to the place of entry to apply the fixing knot), with the thread having to be smooth so that tissues could slide along it.[6,7]

The next stage of our pioneering therefore became the creation of a double-pointed needle with a smooth suturing thread attached to it in the middle, the Aptos Needle. (*access video on usual needle versus Aptos Needle in the online version of this article at:* http://www.plasticsurgery.theclinics.com/) Such a needle is capable of being passed bidirectionally, which allows for it to be passed under the skin along a polygonal or elongated contour, also providing subcutaneous suturing through the soft tissues without dimpling of the skin and obtaining an even lifted contour.

With the help of different Aptos Needle modifications (**Fig. 8**), we worked out minimally invasive aesthetic operations for sewing through soft tissues of the midface, the submaxillary and cervical zones (2003), the chin, elongated and distended lobes of the ear, and ptosed mammary gland (2004).

Sewing Through and Lifting of the Midface

This technique may be used independently and in a combination with the classic or transconjunctival

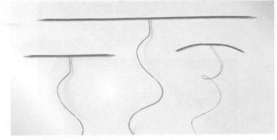

Fig. 8. Different modifications of the Aptos Needle.

blepharoplasty (**Fig. 9**). (*access video on APTOS Needle-midface in the online version of this article at:* http://www.plasticsurgery.theclinics.com/)

In the first instance, the operation commenced from making a 2- to 3-mm cutaneous incision along the lower crow's-foot line, advancing the scalpel's blade to the osseous edge of the eye socket (**Fig. 9**, point 1). This approach was used to introduce the tip of the Aptos Needle 4/0 (from either side) so that it could entrap the periosteum. Then the needle was advanced to point 2 near the base of the wing of the nostril. Here it was carefully brought from under the skin, but not completely, with the second needle's tip remaining within fatty tissues at a depth of 0.5 to 1.0 cm, followed by rotating the Aptos Needle by 90° and then the second needle's tip being advanced toward point 3. Here the needle was also brought to the surface with incomplete exit. Then the needle was rotated 90°, returned to the site of the incision, and brought to the surface through the wound. Here both ends of the thread were pulled and tied by several knots.

The second and third sutures were applied in the similar manner according to the marking. Taken all together they had various direction vectors and created a new, elevated, aesthetically more favorable contour of soft tissues, with smooth transition to the neighboring regions.

For an operation performed through the classic or transconjunctival approach, after isolation and excision of fatty hernias in the amount required, soft tissues of the midface were sutured through so that the knots were distributed along the perimeter of the lower osseous edge of the orbit, arcus marginalis (**Fig. 9**).

To sew through and lift the submaxillary and cervical areas, we made incisions up to 1 cm long from both sides and the retro-aural regions in the projection of the processus mastoideus to the periosteum onto which we applied holding sutures (Prolene 2/0) (**Fig. 10**). (*access video on APTOS Needle-neck in the online version of this article at:* http://www.plasticsurgery.theclinics.com/)

The Aptos Needle 2/0 was inserted through one of the incisions, then advanced subcutaneously along the projection of the lower line of the marking for as long as the length of the thread permitted (usually 15 cm). Here it was brought to surface of the skin and pulled out, but not completely. When the second tip remained under the skin at a depth of approximately 0.5 cm, the needle was turned and the second tip was used to continue passing the thread farther according to the marking. Usually it was necessary to again bring the needle to the surface nearer the angle of the mandible on the opposite side, turn the needle, and continue advancing it again with the first tip until it appeared in the wound contralaterally.

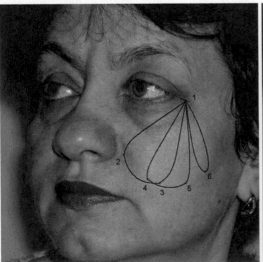
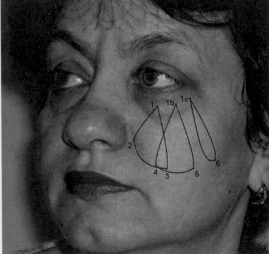

Fig. 9. Marking of midface lifting by the Aptos Needle method.

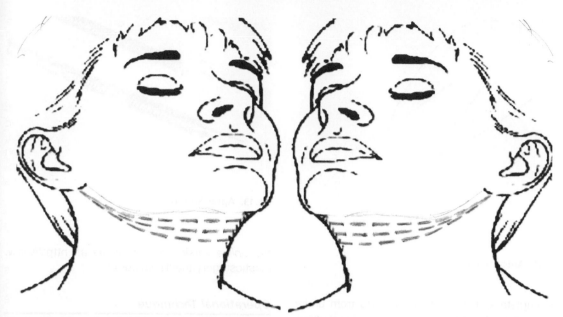

Fig. 10. Marking of neck lifting by the Aptos Needle method.

Here the needle was completely brought to the surface, with the thread pulled out as far as it would go, after having its end preliminarily tied to the holding threads from the first side. At this point the thread was tied to the holding threads on this side.

We performed the same passages of the threaded needle first along the upper and then along the middle lines of the marking, each time tying up to the holding threads on both sides.

Three threads were thus advanced under the skin of the submaxillary region without dimpling of the skin and with anchoring of the ends of the threads to the periosteum of the mastoid processes, like a hammock lifting and supporting soft tissues in a new position, improving the contour of the entire submaxillary and cervical regions. (*access videos on Aptos Needle-chin and Aptos Needle-breast in the online version of this article at:* http://www.plasticsurgery.theclinics.com/)

Aptos Needle 2G Method

Our latest development is experimental so far—the suturing material and Aptos Needle 2G method.[8] (*access video on Aptos Needle 2G in the online version of this article at:* http://www.plasticsurgery.theclinics.com/)

This new product unites the capabilities of Aptos Thread 2G and the Aptos Needle. The Aptos Needle 2G and the Aptos Thread 2G make up one thread with variously directed barbs converging toward the middle and two needles. These needles are double-pointed and the thread is connected to them in the middle portion, as in the Aptos Needle (**Fig. 11**). Like the needles of the Aptos Thread 2G, the tips of the needles of the Aptos Needle 2G are fastened together on one side with temporal soldering, constituting in this position a single tip. This design makes it possible to insert both needles under the skin through one puncture and to separate them at the required depth. Owing to the original idea of coupling two needles, the operations can be done without incision or dimpling of the skin.

The operative procedure using the Aptos Needle 2G method is not more difficult than manipulations with the Aptos Thread 2G, but lifting of soft tissues herein is more powerful and stable at the expense of subcutaneous turns of the needle and advancing the barbed thread along the contour of the "pouch" or a hook without disturbing the integrity of bulges and dimpling of the skin. We used the product and technique of the operation Aptos Needle 2G on virtually all portions of the face to move tissues and to create high contours; however, so far we can recommend it for wide application only in lifting of the midface zone (**Fig. 12**).

The operation was performed approximately in the same manner as the Aptos Thread 2G technique: the twin needle was inserted into the area of the zygomatic arch, to be separated in the subcutaneous fat at a depth of approximately 1 cm around the portion of the fascial bands, and the thread was advanced farther on each needle according to the marking. After exiting and

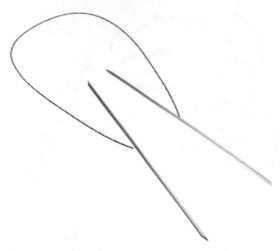

Fig. 11. Aptos Needle 2G.

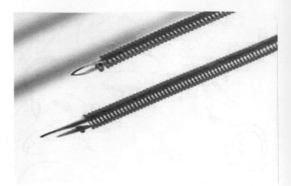

Fig. 13. Aptos Springs.

incomplete surfacing of the needles from under the skin they were turned within subcutaneous fat (as with the usual Aptos Needle) and along a new contour returned back to the area of the zygomatic arch, where after moderate pulling the threads were cut and the ends submerged under the derma.

Aptos Spring Method

Involutive alterations in the kinetically active zones (marionette lines, ptosis of the angles of the mouth) were removed by the elastic lifting with special threads[9] we devised in 2003. This is a heliciform thread made according to a special technology from special shape-memory POLYPROPYLENE (**Fig. 13**). (*access video on Aptos Spring in*

the online version of this article at: http://www. plasticsurgery.theclinics.com/)

Operational Technique

To lift marionette lines, it is necessary to implant two Aptos Spring threads on each side perpendicular to the wrinkle itself (**Fig. 14**). Because the spring needle is coiled onto an aspirating needle and is thus in a compressed state, before being applied it was freed from fixation on the side of the base and spread along the needle's length. In this working condition of the spring, the needle was inserted in the area of the zygomatic arch, advanced subcutaneously according to the marking, and surfaced approximately 1 cm after passing of the tip of the wrinkle's projection. Then the thread was released from fixation from the side of the tip, with the surgeon slightly pulling the ends of the spring and cutting off the extra

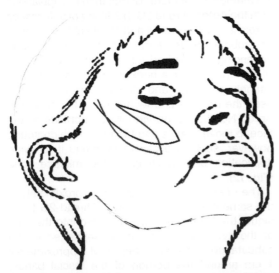

Fig. 12. Marking of lifting by the Aptos Needle 2G method.

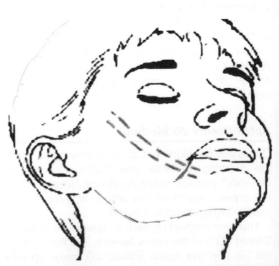

Fig. 14. Marking of lifting by the Aptos Springs method.

length, submerging the ends under the skin. Other threads were placed in a similar manner.

To lift the angles of the mouth, the upper thread was implanted in a somewhat different manner to the angle of the mouth and farther along the projection of the vermilion border of the upper lip by approximately 1 to 1.5 cm. Doing so made it possible to slightly invert the lateral edge of the upper lip to somehow increase its volume and to attain an alteration in the direction of the angle of the mouth upwards.

RESULTS AND DISCUSSION

Of the 4580 patients, 2133 underwent the manipulation as an independent operation. In the rest it was done in combination with other operations and procedures, including undercutting of wrinkles and folds (Aptos Wire method), autolifting, liposuction of mental, submaxillary, and cervical regions, facial skin peeling, blepharoplasty, face lift, platysmaplasty (**Fig. 15**), and others. **Figs. 16–20** show patients who underwent simultaneous operations.

In most cases we used infiltration anesthesia consisting of 1% lidocaine solution with epinephrine; the solution was injected while the threads were placed, with an average of 0.3 to 0.5 mL of the solution used for one thread. Anesthetics were used in greater amounts only during the operation of lifting the submaxillary and cervical areas by the Aptos Needle method. In that procedure the percentage of the anesthetic was decreased to 0.5 or 0.25.

Among our patients, we observed age-related ptosis of the involutional pattern more often and saw acquired ptosis resulting from disease or iatrogenic causes less frequently (a total of 38 patients). We saw congenital ptosis in separate cases (11 patients).

Typically, operations using the Aptos methods proceeded easily and quickly, with the injury inflicted to tissues being minimal and the outcome of the intervention seen as early as on the operative table.

The Aptos methods are especially effective in the midface zone: the nasolabial fold becomes uncrumpled, the lachrymal fold is smoothed out, and the soft tissues are elevated and moved upward and laterally, thus creating an integral, even round contour of the buccozygomatic area. Based on follow-up of patients over several years, we noted preservation of good outcomes from 1 year and more in most, with the best effect being achieved after implantation of the threads Aptos Needle and Aptos Needle 2G (**Figs. 21–25**). Complete relapses of the deformity in the region concerned were observed only in sporadic cases.

In the area of the tail of the eyebrow (Aptos Thread 2G), we obtained pronounced lifting upward and laterally, and moderate spreading of the upper eyelid skin, especially in the lateral portion. Immediately after surgery, extra lifting of the eyebrow and goffered skin in the area of the temple was considered justified, because within the first 2 to 3 weeks during the period of stabilization of the clinical result, skin adaptation and slight lowering of the brow occurred. We were satisfied if

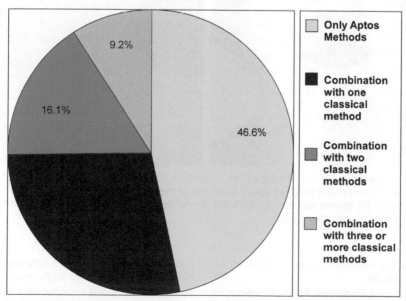

Fig.15. For 2133 of the 4580 patients, the manipulation was performed as an independent operation. In the rest it was done in a combination with one or more classic methods.

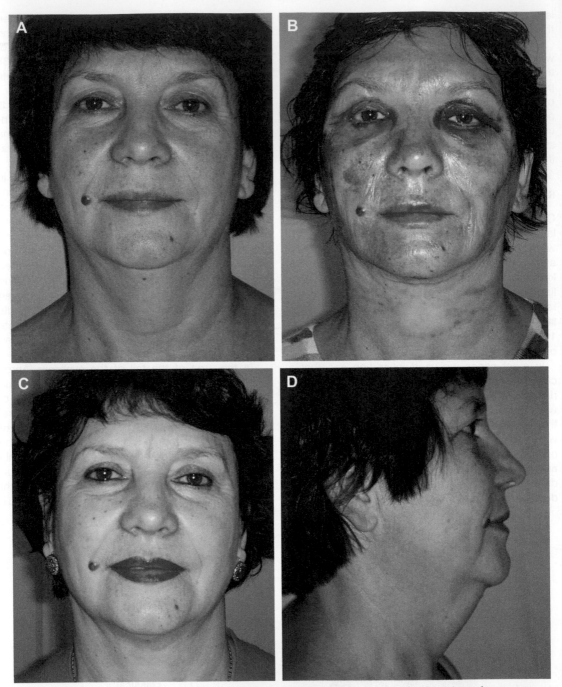

Fig. 16. (*A, D*) A 52-year-old patient is shown before surgery. (*B, E*) The patient is shown 3 days after surgery consisting of upper and lower classic blepharoplasty, stitching of the midface by Aptos Needle, lifting of the mental area by Aptos Thread 2G, liposuction of the submaxillary and cervical area, and Aptos Needle stitching. (*C, F*) The same patient is shown 1 year after surgery.

the good outcome obtained persisted for 8 to 12 months (**Figs. 26–29**).

In the mental area (methods Aptos Thread and Aptos Thread 2G), depending on the degree of ptosis and skin excess after the operation, we observed more or less pronounced lifting of hanging lips and skin redistribution upward and laterally. We noted wrinkled skin in the immediate postoperative period on the background of pronounced improvement of the oval of the face.

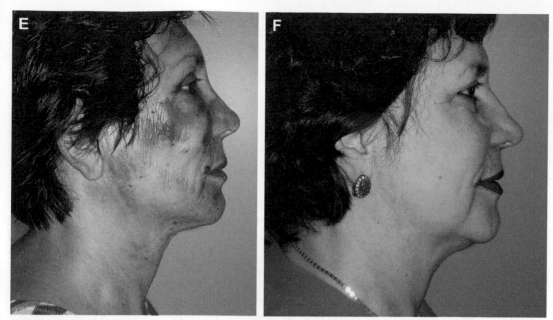

Fig. 16. (continued).

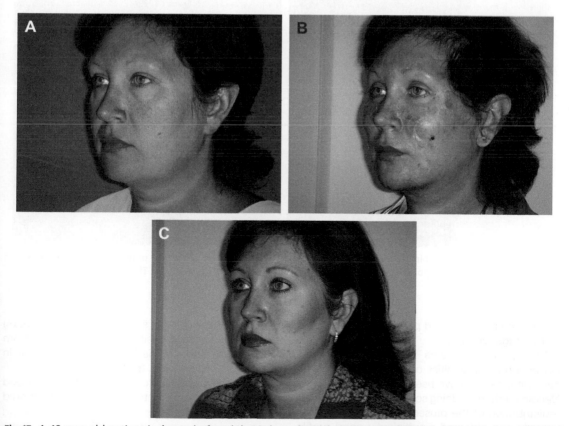

Fig. 17. A 48-year-old patient is shown before (A), 10 days after (B), and 11 months after (C) surgery consisting of upper and lower classic blepharoplasty, stitching of the midface by Aptos Needle, liposuction of the submaxillary and cervical area, and Aptos Needle stitching.

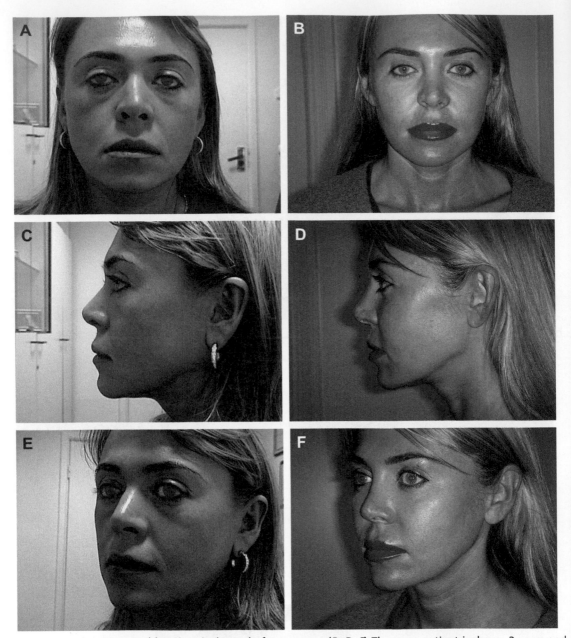

Fig. 18. (*A, C, E*) A 37-year-old patient is shown before surgery. (*B, D, F*) The same patient is shown 2 years and 7 months after face autolipofilling, and midface and mental area lifting by Aptos Thread.

In most cases, we noted persistent results up to 1 year (**Figs. 30, 31**).

During the last years for minimally invasive correction of deformities of the submaxillary and cervical area, we have been using only the Aptos Needle method. In doing so, we attained moderate redistribution of the ptosed skin from the middle laterally and obtained a sufficiently good profile. We observed no complete relapse of the deformity even after 3 to 4 years. Certain weakening of the

threads and sagging of soft tissues (after 1–3 years) were, if necessary, easily corrected by lifting from one of the ends of the knot and anchoring it in a higher position (**Figs. 32–34**).

The success factors for obtaining good outcomes while using the Aptos methods of rigid fixation are as follows:

Use only when indicated and correctly select the method.

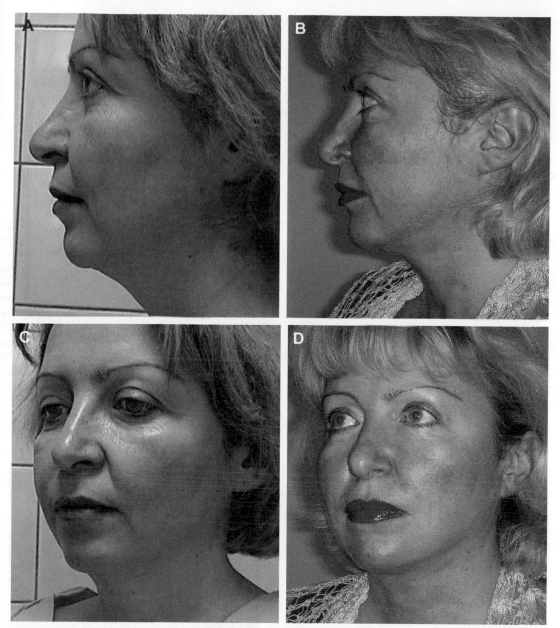

Fig.19. (*A, C*) A 45-year-old patient is shown before surgery. (*B, D*) The patient is shown 2 years and 8 months after upper and lower classic blepharoplasty, stitching of the midface by Aptos Needle, liposuction of the submaxillary and cervical area, Aptos Needle stitching, marionette lines lifting by Aptos Springs, and browlift by Aptos Thread 2G.

Determine the purpose of the operation (ie, what effect is expected from the implantation of the threads) lifting of tissues, their redistribution, creation of a new high volume, or a combination of these effects.

Place the threads in areas where they cannot counteract the kinetics of facial muscles and where you can easily remove layers of soft tissues unimpeded without operative dissection thereof.

Observe the depth for placing the threads depending on the purposes of the operation, the condition of the skin, and the portion of the face.

Place the threads such that the barbs from each side of the thread are equal both quantitatively and by strength (this condition concerns only Aptos Thread).

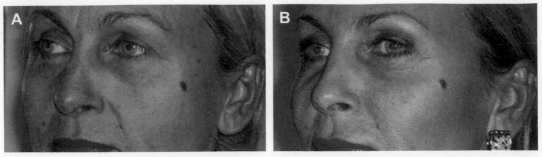

Fig. 20. A 53-year-old patient is shown before (A) and 17 months after (B) midface lifting by Aptos Thread.

All the above-described types of thread-mediated lifting are rigid. On the areas of the face that are especially active (for example, mimic, masticatory, and other muscles in the perioral area), lifting with barbed threads or by the Aptos Needle method is unsuitable because constant tissue movement rapidly destroys the result. For correction of involutive alterations in the perioral area we therefore used the Aptos Spring method.

In virtually all cases, this technique allowed removal of labiosubmaxillary wrinkles and provided nonrigid, elastic lifting of the angles of the mouth in the immediate and remote postoperative periods. Polypropylene springs placed in subcutaneous fat in the distended form contract and delicately entail the soft tissues. They contract and extend synchronously with the muscles during the mimic and masticatory movements. Several months after, the threads are covered with fibrous tissue, which later enhances and stabilizes the effect. With the exception of several cases of a rapid relapse of the deformity, when the contracting springs were not fixed in tissues but slipped into the needle-created channel, we observed a stable outcome within 1 to 2 years (**Figs. 35–38**).

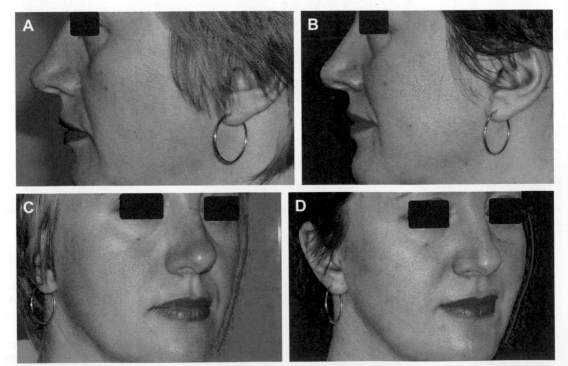

Fig. 21. (A, C) A 36-year-old patient of is shown before surgery. (B, D) The patient is shown 2 years after midface lifting by Aptos Thread.

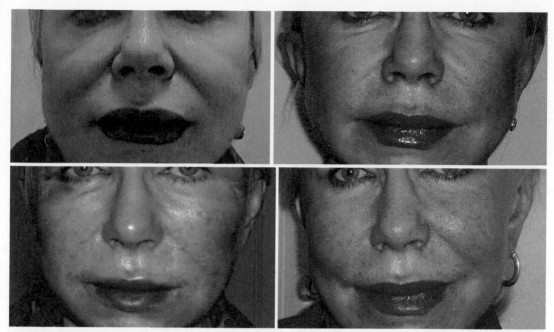

Fig. 22. A 54-year-old patient is shown before surgery (*upper left*). The same patient is shown 5 days after midface stitching by Aptos Needle (*lower left*), 18 months later (*upper right*), and 3 years and 6 months later (*lower right*).

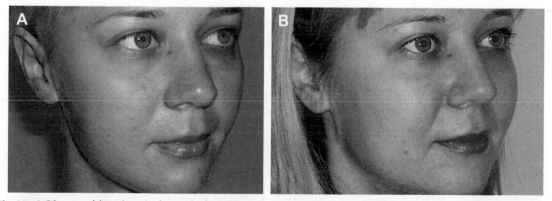

Fig. 23. A 29-year-old patient is shown before (*A*) and 3 years and 3 months after (*B*) midface stitching by Aptos Needle through a transconjunctival blepharoplasty approach.

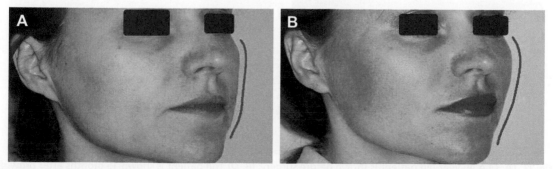

Fig. 24. A 37-year-old patient is shown before (*A*) and 11 months after (*B*) midface Aptos Thread 2G.

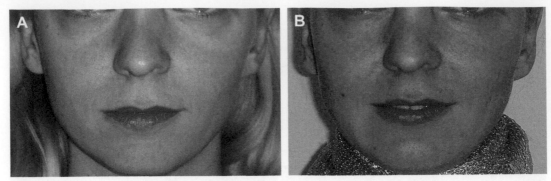

Fig. 25. A 35-year-old patient is shown before (*A*) and 13 months after (*B*) midface lift by Aptos Thread 2G.

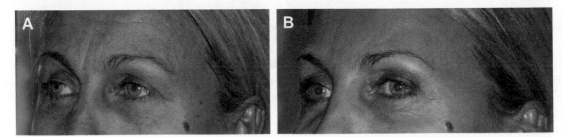

Fig. 26. A 53-year-old patient is shown before (*A*) and 17 months after (*B*) browlift by Aptos Thread 2G.

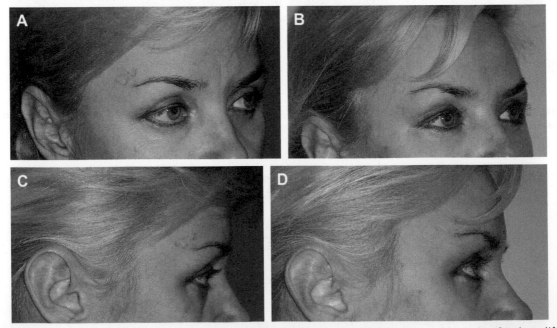

Fig. 27. (*A, C*) A 46-year-old patient is shown before surgery. (*B, D*) The patient is shown 15 months after browlift by Aptos Thread 2G.

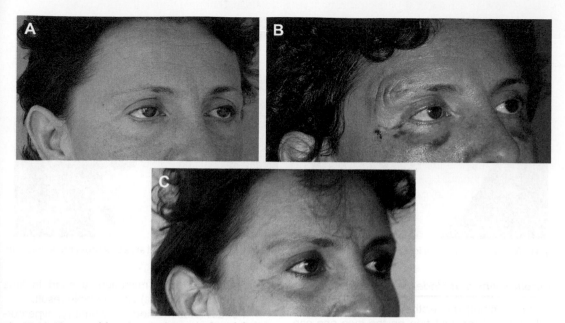

Fig. 28. A 40-year-old patient is shown before (*A*), 3 days after (*B*), and 11 months after (*C*) brow-tail lift by Aptos Thread 2G.

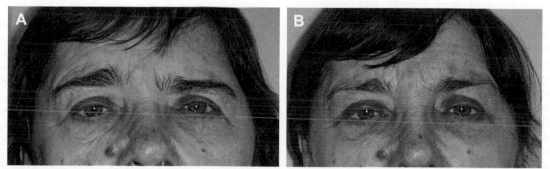

Fig. 29. (*A*) A 67-year-old patient is shown after transection of the rami temporales nervi facialis face lift. She is pictured before surgery. (*B*) The same patient is shown 8 months after left-side browlift by Aptos Thread 2G.

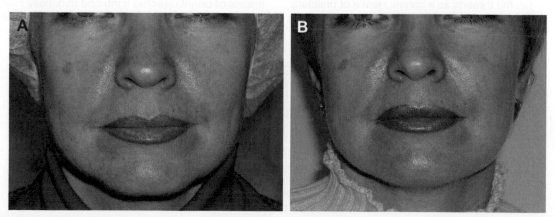

Fig. 30. A 44-year-old patient is shown before (*A*) and 1 year after (*B*) lifting of the mental area by Aptos Thread 2G.

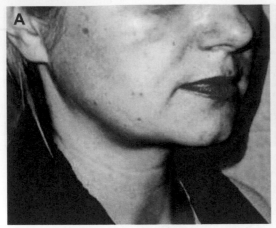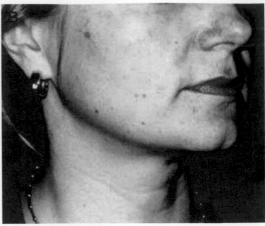

Fig. 31. A 38-year-old patient is shown before (*A*) and 5 months after (*B*) lifting of mental area by Aptos Thread method.

Complications and Undesirable Events

While performing any aesthetic operation or minimally invasive manipulation on the face one can encounter complications, such as inflammatory processes up to suppuration; disturbed integrity of the parotid salivary gland, little branches of the facial nerve or large vessels; and hematomas. The Aptos methods are not guaranteed against such complications.[10–12] Such complications are not intrinsic to the nature of the method itself. Prevention of the mentioned complications consists of observing the principles of the regional anatomy of the face and its peculiarities, using asepsis and antiseptics, delicately performing an intervention, and treatment, including antibacterial therapy, general surgical intervention, and special intervention (microsurgical, physiotherapeutic, and others) (**Figs. 39, 40**).

Characteristic of the methods of thread-mediated lifting and side effects are as follows:

> For the Aptos Thread method: disruption of the threads as a consequence of unilateral slackening of the barbs, surfacing of the

threads, their migration, a short in time (up to 3 months) and unstable result.

For all Aptos methods: asymmetry, hypercorrection, visualization of the threads, linear hemorrhages along the length of the thread, hematomas, and dimpling of the skin in the site of needle punctures (**Figs. 41–46**).

Prevention of the mentioned complications, side effects, and undesirable events consists of knowing the pathogenesis of ageing and ptosis of the facial soft tissues, correct understanding of the essence of lifting by the Aptos methods and selecting the proper method, faultless handling of the technique, and delicate performance of the intervention. Treatment is associated with removal of the slackened and migrating threads, repeat thread-mediated or classic lifting, physiotherapy, and massage.

For thread removal in our clinic we use the methods of noninvasive detection of threads under the skin (ultrasonography, visualization by means of bright directed light) and minimally invasive removal thereof by means of a special needle.

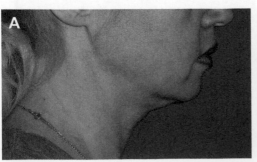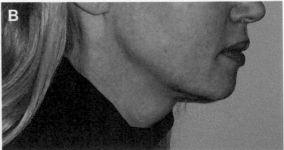

Fig. 32. A 46-year-old patient is shown before (*A*) and 15 months after (*B*) stitching of the submaxillary and cervical areas by Aptos Needle.

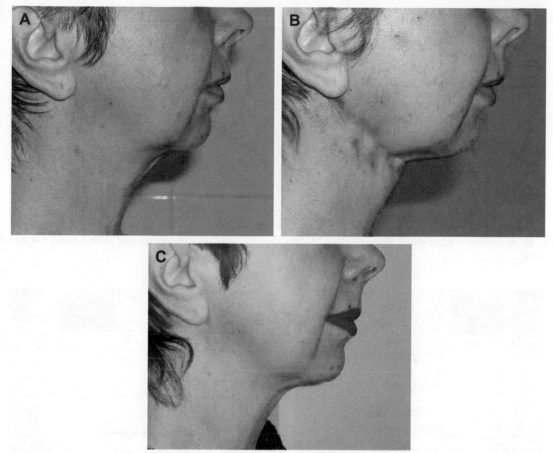

Fig. 33. A 55-year-old patient is shown before (*A*), 4 days after (*B*), and 18 months after (*C*) stitching of the submaxillary and cervical areas by Aptos Needle.

With experience, this manipulation presents no difficulty for the operator (**Fig. 47**).

Complications and unfavorable events are so rare and inconsiderable that specialists in aesthetic surgery and cosmetology should not abandon the methods of thread-mediated lifting for this reason.

As we have gained experience in using the Aptos methods, we have been constantly improving them, enhancing the power of lifting, the safety

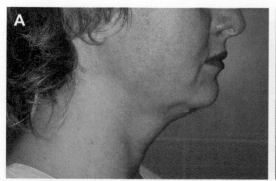
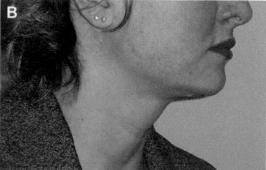

Fig. 34. A 35-year-old patient is shown before (*A*) and 15 months after (*B*) stitching of the submaxillary and cervical areas with the Aptos Needle.

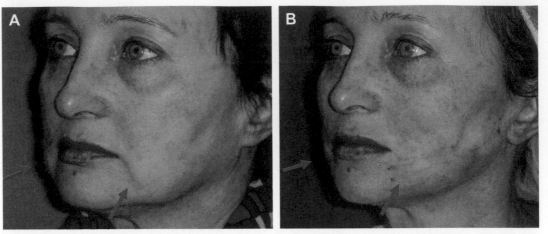

Fig. 35. A 43-year-old patient is shown before (*A*) and directly after (*B*) marionette line lifting using the Aptos Spring.

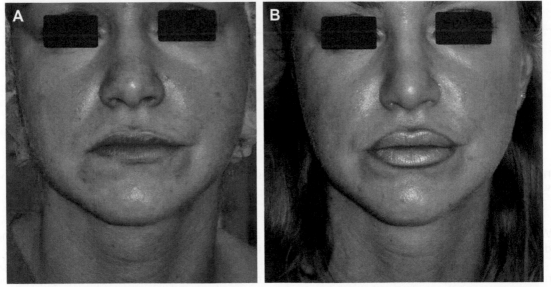

Fig. 36. A 35-year-old patient with right-side phlegmon of the upper jaw is shown before (*A*) and 3 months after (*B*) right-side lifting of the angle of the mouth using the Aptos Spring.

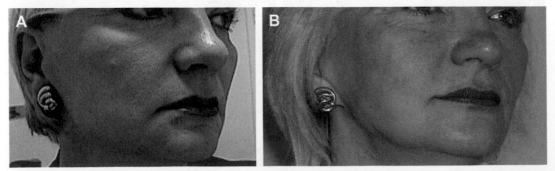

Fig. 37. A 60-year-old patient is shown before (*A*) and 20 months after (*B*) marionette line lifting using the Aptos Spring.

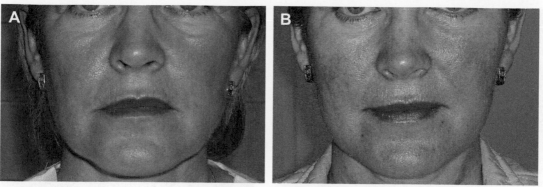

Fig. 38. A 46-year-old patient is shown before (*A*) and 4 months after (*B*) marionette line lifting using the Aptos Spring and midface lifting with Aptos Thread.

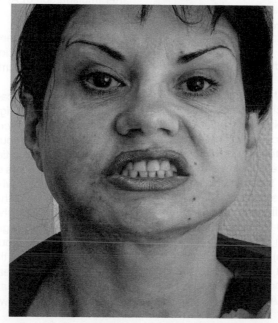

Fig. 39. Two days after implantation of Aptos Thread, this patient had hematoma of the mental and buccal areas.

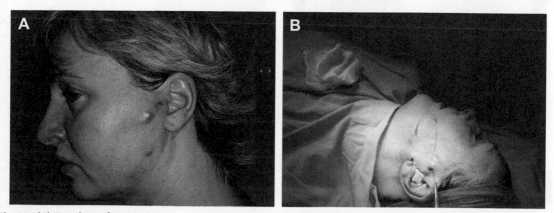

Fig. 40. (*A*) Ten days after implantation of Aptos Thread 2G, the patient had suppuration of the thread insertion site. (*B*) The moment of thread removal is shown.

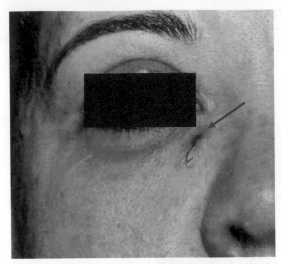

Fig. 41. This patient had thread migration 4 months after implantation of Aptos Thread.

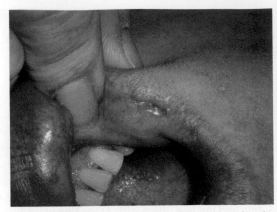

Fig. 43. Superficial arrangement of thread under the mucous membrane was seen in this patient 3 months after implantation of Aptos Springs.

of the operation, and the durability and stability of the results.

We have experienced all things characteristic of implementing any novel technologies: initial admiration and euphoria, disappointments, complications, and cautious attitude. Because of these circumstances and because doctors of our clinic are the designers of the Aptos methods we can express our opinion concerning thread-mediated lifting methods suggested by other authors.

Many doctors have still been placing barbed threads using an outdated technique that requires incisions and visualization of solid structures (for example, temporal fascia) to which threads are sewn. With the advent of coupled needles provided with threads and the respective technology (methods using Aptos Thread 2G and

Aptos Needle 2G), there is no need for skin incisions, and the operations are thus considerably simplified with no damage for the future result (**Fig. 48**).[13]

We doubt the efficacy of using long barbed threads for lifting and rigid fixation of the kinetically active zones of the face and neck, and the feasibility of their use without taking into consideration the anatomic peculiarities of various facial regions (**Fig. 48**B). The authors of this methodology do not explain, for instance, what happens to the threads' barbs directed from the temporal or even bregmatic areas through the entire cheek downward to the submaxillary region, when a person widely opens his or her mouth. Also unclear is what happens to threads that have been advanced from the temporal area downward to the upper lip (the nasolabial triangle), to the labiomental fold (marionette line) when the patient produces

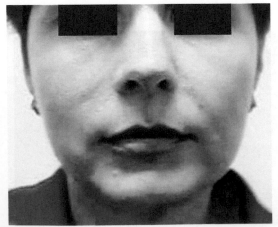

Fig. 42. This patient had asymmetry 1 week after implantation of Aptos Thread.

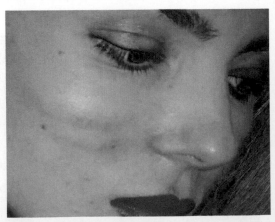

Fig. 44. Superficial arrangement of thread under the skin was seen in this patient 2.5 months after implantation of Aptos Thread.

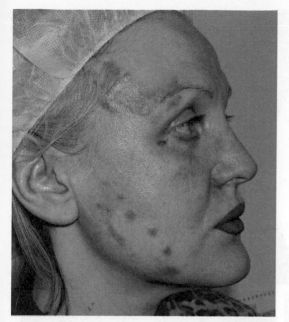

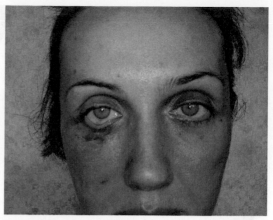

Fig. 46. The patient is shown 2 weeks after lower blepharoplasty and midface stitching by the Aptos Needle. One of the stitches is sewed to the edge of the eyelid, not to the periosteum of the arcus marginalis.

Fig. 45. This patient had an allergic reaction 2 days after implantation of Aptos Thread.

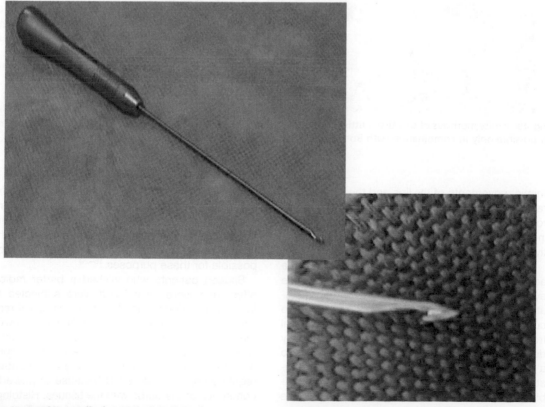

Fig. 47. Furrier needle for removing threads.

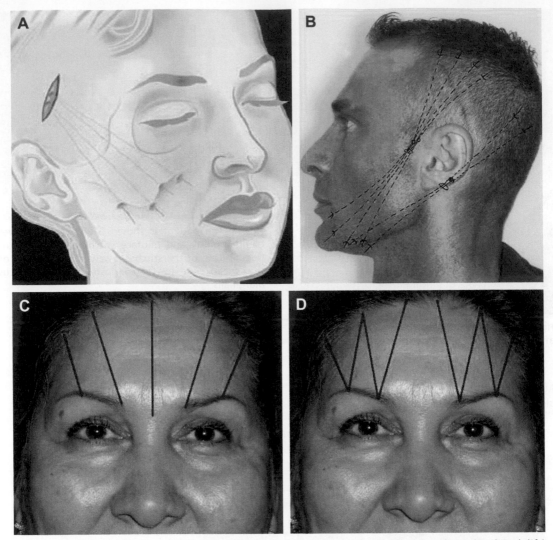

Fig. 48. Faulty methods of soft tissue lifting by threads with protrusions. (*A, B*) Wrong marking. (*C, D*) Such lifting is possible only in combination with Botox injections.

mimic movements of the lips and the entire perio-ral area. Procedures placing threads from the ret-roaural area to the submental and cervical regions in the form of a fan also usually prove to be ineffec-tive (**Fig. 48**B).[14]

We also do not recommend following the advice of those colleagues who lift the whole eyebrow and even the forehead by thread-medi-ated methods.[15] Doing so, they do not take into consideration the presence of the powerful frontal muscle and its kinetics, which rapidly destroy the barbs of the threads, leading to a relapse of the deformity (**Fig. 48**C). In this situ-ation it seems appropriate to study the possi-bility of simultaneously using the Aptos Needle 2G method and Botox.

During endoscopic face lift procedures for sewing through the ptosed tissues, many surgeons use suture material that is inconvenient for this purpose and that leaves dimpling on the skin. The Aptos Needle is the best method possible for these purposes.[16–20]

Sixteen patients who wished a better radical effect and were dissatisfied were subjected to face lift at various times following the first thread lifting (0.5–2 years). Intraoperative findings showed that the implanted threads were in those sites where they had been placed. Neither their color nor their structure was altered, and their removal required considerable effort because of powerful coherence of the barbs with the tissues. Histology revealed that within tissues, the Aptos Threads

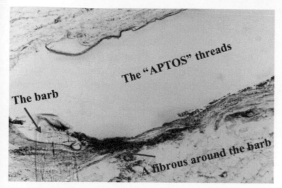

Fig. 49. Morphologic specimen eventuated by face lift (1 year after implantation of Aptos Thread).

were covered with a solid fibrous membrane, which was especially pronounced around the barbs, which is yet another explanation of the cause of stability and persistence of good clinical results (**Fig. 49**).[21,22]

SUMMARY

Absolute advantages of using the Aptos technologies while performing lifting are as follows:

Simplicity, easiness, economy of use
Minimally invasive nature and low trauma of the procedures
Reliability and sufficient duration of qualitative lifting
Possible combination with other interventions and a short rehabilitation period

The Aptos methods constitute a new, nontraditional trend in aesthetic surgery, requiring further study and development. Despite the apparent simplicity, these operations do have their own nuances, which if taken into consideration and complied with provide a good stable outcome.

Unskillful hands and insufficient experience could at best yield undesirable results and rapid relapses and at worst complications. Such practitioners would rapidly be disappointed, ascribing failures to imperfection of the method and speaking against it, which is unfortunate. Doing so, they ignore suggestions to undergo a teaching course. These circumstances thwart progress and hamper improvement not only of the Aptos method but also of minimally invasive aesthetic surgery as a whole. To dismiss suture lifting gives no chance to a large number of patients who have appropriate indications and the desire to rejuvenate their appearance to have an alternative to the classic method of lifting and contour plasty of the face.

APPENDIX: SUPPLEMENTARY MATERIAL

Supplementary material can be found, in the online version, at doi:10.1016/j.cps.2008.12.003.

REFERENCES

1. Kazinnikova OG, Adamian AA. Age-specific changes in facial and cervical tissues, a review. Ann Plast Rec Aest Surg (Rus.) 2000;1:52–61.
2. Mendelson BC, Muzaffar AR, Adams WP, et al. Surgical anatomy of the midcheek and malar mounds, plastic and reconstructive surgery 2002;110(N3):885–96.
3. Sulamanidze MA, Fournier PF, Paikidze TG, et al. Removal of facial soft tissue ptosis with special threads. Dermatol Surg 2002;28:367–71.
4. Frischberg IA. Face aesthetic surgery. ICC "Akademkniga", 2005. p. 271.
5. Sulamanidze M, Paikidze T, Sulamanidze G, et al. Utilisation du fil «APTOS» dans le lifting facial. La Revue De Chirurgie Esthetique de Langue Francaise 2001;25(103):17–22.
6. Sulamanidze MA, Sulamanidze GM. Flabby, ageing face. A new approach. II Congress on aesthetic and restorative surgery, Moscow1998. p. 15.
7. Fournier P. Les variants dans la technique du Curl Lift, La revue de chirurgie esthetique de langue Francaise. t. XXVIII, n 2004;117:35–8.
8. Sulamanidze M, Sulamanidze G. Lifting of soft tissues: old philosophy, new approach—a method of internal stitching (Aptos needle). J Japan Society Aesthetic Surg 2005;42(5):182.
9. Sulamanidze M, Sulamanidze G. Surgical suture material and a method to the use thereof, WO 2007/133103 A1.
10. Sulamanidze M, Sulamanidze G. APTOS SPRING—a new concept of lifting. J Japan Society Aesthetic Surg 2005;42(5):183.
11. Sulamanidze M, Sulamanidze G. Aptos threads, side effects, complications APTOS. Congreso International de dermatilogia cosmetica. 3 al 5 de Julio del Ciudad de Mexico 2003.
12. Helling ER, Okpaku A, Wang PH, et al. Complications of facial suspension sutures. Aesthet Surg J 2007;27(2):155–61.
13. Winkler E, Goldan O, Regev E, et al. Stensen duct rupture (sialocele) and other complications of the Aptos thread technique. Plast Reconstr Surg 2006;118:1468–71.
14. Aesthetic buyers guide.www.miinews.com; 2006.
15. Guillo D. Fils Aptos implantation en X. Surginevs, Automne 2005;8:10.
16. Woffles Wu. Advances in stitch lift. 2nd regional conference in dermatological laser and facial cosmetic surgery 2006 20–22 January, Hong Kong, Programme Book, p. 30
17. Isse N. Endiscopic facial rejuvenation: endoforehead, the functional lift. Aesthetic Plast Surg 1994;18:21–9.

18. Ramirez OM. Endoscopic subperiosteal browlift and facelift. Clin Plast Surg 1995;22:639–60.

19. Freeman SM. Transconjunctival sub-orbicularis oculi fat (SOOF) Pad lift blepharoplasty. Arch Facial Plast Surg 2000;2:16–21.

20. Little JW. Three dimensional rejuvenation of the midface: volumetric resculpture by malar imbrication. Plast Reconstr Surg 2000;105(1): 267–85.

21. Fuente del Campo A. Update on minimally invasive face lift technique. Aesthet Surg J 2008;28:51–61.

22. Adamyan A, Skuba N, Sulamanidze M, et al. Morphological foundations of facelift using APTOS filaments. Ann Plast Reconstr Aesthetic Surg (RU) 2002;3:19–27.

A New Approach for the Prophylactic Improvement of Surgical Scarring: Avotermin (TGFβ3)

V. Leroy Young, MD[a],*, James Bush, MBChB, MRCS (Ed)[b],
Sharon O'Kane, PhD[b]

KEYWORDS

- Avotermin • Transforming growth factor β3
- Cicatrix • Scarring • Surgery

PATIENTS ARE CONCERNED ABOUT SCARRING FROM ELECTIVE AND AESTHETIC SURGICAL PROCEDURES

Scarring following aesthetic plastic surgery is a major issue for surgeons and their patients. The authors recently collaborated in a research survey investigating concerns about scarring in two groups:[1] United States patients who recently had undergone a routine surgical procedure (97 in total) and[2] plastic and dermatological surgeons conducting aesthetic procedures (24 in total). The survey confirmed that patients and clinicians are concerned with surgical scars and that patients in particular value any opportunity to improve or minimize scarring.[3] Overall, 60% of patients were dissatisfied with scars resulting from their recent surgery, with similar rates of dissatisfaction seen in patients with different gender, age, and ethnicity. Although the patients surveyed indicated that they were concerned with scars on visible body sites, they also identified scar(s) over a range of body sites (visible and nonvisible) that they wished were less noticeable. Data from the survey raised questions about the accuracy of gender stereotypes on the acceptability of scarring. Although half (48%) of the patients said that it is acceptable for a man to have a scar, only 25% thought that it was acceptable for a woman to have a scar. When patients were asked about their own scars, however, a very different picture emerged. Most (greater than 90%) of both men and women indicated that they wished their own scars were less noticeable, and more than one third of men admitted that they had tried to conceal their scar.

The clinician survey showed that plastic surgeons and aesthetic dermatologists have a high awareness of patients' concerns, with 96% agreeing that scarring was a concern for most of their patients and 100% agreeing that they always attempt to prevent/improve scarring when conducting a surgical procedure. The surveys, however, revealed issues in the communication between patients and clinicians regarding scars. The survey showed that most patients had expected the scar resulting from their recent surgical procedure to be less noticeable than it was, but only 64% of patients had discussed the

Dr. Young has received research funding and honorarium payments from Renovo, the biotechnology company undertaking the clinical development of avotermin. Dr. Bush is Head of Surgery, and Dr. O'Kane is chief scientific officer of Renovo; both of these authors also own shares in Renovo.
[a] BodyAesthetic Plastic Surgery and Skincare Center, 969 North Mason Road, Suite 170, St. Louis, MO 63141, USA
[b] Renovo Ltd., 48 Grafton Street, Manchester, M13 9XX, UK
* Corresponding author.
E-mail address: leroyyoungmd@bodyaesthetic.com (V.L. Young).

Clin Plastic Surg 36 (2009) 307–313
doi:10.1016/j.cps.2008.11.008
0094-1298/08/$ – see front matter © 2009 Elsevier Inc. All rights reserved.

possibility of scarring with their surgeon. Overall, 71% of patients agreed that they were more concerned with scarring than their surgeon, and 60% said that their surgeon could be more sensitive to how they felt about their scar from a recent surgical procedure. Patients were very sensitive and valued any opportunity to improve scars. Overall, 91% agreed that even a small improvement in scarring on a visible site would be worthwhile. To address patients' expectations about scarring, surgeons need to clearly communicate the possibility and severity of scarring following surgery, and demonstrate that they are doing all that is possible to reduce scarring, irrespective of how small the final scar might be.

The management of patients' expectations about scarring following aesthetic procedures is a complex area. The perceived severity of a surgical scar is influenced by three dimensions (**Fig. 1**):

- The surgical technique undertaken (and, of course, the expertise of the surgeon)
- The objective appearance of the scar (influenced by a range of biological and wound factors)
- The overall impact of the scar on the patient

The impact of the scar can be related to impairment of function and physical symptoms such as chronic pain and itching. The sensitivity of the patient to the scar is a major factor influencing the perception of severity, however. Objectively, the noticeability of a scar depends on how closely it blends with surrounding normal skin, both in the short and longer term. Studies and the authors' clinical experience, however, indicate that patients' anxiety and self-consciousness about their scars do not correlate with the severity of the scar.[1,2,4] One patient with a relatively minor

scar may suffer as much anxiety as another with a severely disfiguring scar. Patient sensitivity can be influenced by the cause of the scar and whether it is the legacy of a traumatic event or illness. Scar location is another factor influencing patient sensitivity, as it determines whether the scar is visible. Visible, however, is also a subjective concept that varies according to social situation (eg, a scar that is not visible in a professional context may be revealed during sport or leisure activities). In the patient survey discussed previously, scars on a range of body sites (both visible and nonvisible) caused patients concern, and nearly one third of patients indicated that they would be embarrassed to have a scar that was seen only by their partner. Demographics and the cultural context of the patient also have a major influence on sensitivity to scarring, particularly in societies where there is pressure to conform to an idealized appearance.

SCARRING IN THE MODERN SURGICAL CONTEXT

The optimal outcome of wound repair is the complete restoration of normal (unwounded) skin architecture, strength, and function. The major evolutionary forces shaping the cellular and molecular mechanisms underlying adult wound healing were directed at walling off foreign bodies and infectious agents, and rapidly replacing missing tissue with partly functioning repair tissue (ie, a scar). This response was driven by wounds with variable amounts of tissue damage that were exposed to dirty conditions, such as would be encountered in a primitive bite, blow, or other trauma. In this context, speed of healing was balanced against restoration of function so as to preserve the life of the animal.[5] These are not the kinds of wounds most commonly encountered today, however. Today, the most common injuries are those occurring during surgical repair, which involve sharp injuries made under sterile conditions with close approximation of the wound margins. The healing of surgical wounds to the skin has not been optimized by evolutionary forces and, within the modern surgical context, scarring can be considered an inappropriate response.

There is a high unmet need for therapies that are effective for reducing scarring following surgery. The latest statistics from the American Society of Plastic Surgeons show that almost 12 million cosmetic and 5.1 million reconstructive plastic surgery procedures were performed in the United States in 2007.[6] Statistics also reveal that there is a high demand for scar revision, which was the third most frequent reconstructive procedure conducted in the United States in 2007. When

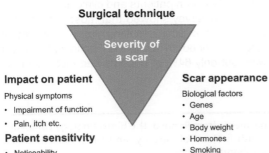

Surgical technique

Severity of a scar

Impact on patient

Physical symptoms
- Impairment of function
- Pain, itch etc.

Patient sensitivity
- Noticeability
  – short and long term
- Cause
- Location
- Demographics

Scar appearance

Biological factors
- Genes
- Age
- Body weight
- Hormones
- Smoking

Wound factors
- Type of injury
- Location
- Mechanical factors
- Wound complications

Fig. 1. Three dimensions affecting the perceived severity of a surgical scar by a patient.

considered in the context of patient concerns about scarring, these statistics clearly identify scarring as an area of high and, as yet, not suitably met medical need. Although several treatments and regimens are used for scar management in clinical practice, no single therapy has been adopted universally in clinical practice.[7–10] This reflects the fact that current treatments used in clinical practice tend to have unclear benefits, resulting in unpredictable, limited, and variable effectiveness. Another major limitation of this therapeutic area is that, generally, treatments have not been evaluated in prospective and sufficiently robust randomized clinical trials.[11]

In recent years, translational research into the processes involved in scarring at the molecular, cellular, and tissue levels has facilitated the discovery and development of new biological approaches for improving scarring. These studies have led to a new concept for scar management, which is the prophylactic improvement of scarring by pharmaceutical agents that are given at the time of surgery to reduce subsequent scar formation (**Table 1**). This prophylactic approach aligns with current clinical practice and will complement current strategies used for the clinical management of scarring. The first in the new class of prophylactic regenerative medicines to enter clinical development was avotermin (also known as Juvista), which is the clinical application of recombinant human transforming growth factor β3 (TGFβ3).

THE ROLE OF TRANSFORMING GROWTH FACTOR β3 IN FETAL SCAR-FREE HEALING

The initial observations leading to the discovery of TGFβ3 came from developmental biology studies evaluating the use of sheep fetuses as surgical models of cleft lip.[5] The studies revealed that, at birth, a wound made to the lip of a sheep fetus between gestational days 60 and 90 healed not only without a scar, but with regeneration of tissue at the macroscopic and microscopic levels. These observations then allowed the study of the molecular, biochemical, and cellular correlates of scar-free versus scar-forming healing, and led to identification of key molecules and pathways associated with these different phenotypes. The TGFβ family of molecules, in particular, was shown to play a central role.[5,12–15] The TGFβ1 and TGFβ2 isoforms were expressed highly in adult wounds that healed with a scar and were either absent or expressed at low levels in embryonic wounds that healed without a scar (**Fig. 2**). Conversely, the TGFβ3 isoform was expressed at high levels in embryonic wounds that healed without a scar. In adult wounds that healed with a scar, TGFβ3 was expressed at a lower level and at a later stage of the healing process compared with the TGFβ1 and TGFβ2 isoforms.

Subsequent studies confirmed that the TGFβ family, TGFβ3 in particular, plays a central role in scar-free healing in the embryo, and suggested that modulation of the levels of TGFβ3 relative to those of TGFβ1 in adults may result in reduced scarring.[16–19] This was confirmed first by studies in a rat cutaneous incisional wound model of scarring, which demonstrated that neutralization of the profibrotic molecules TGFβ1 and TGFβ2 by the addition of antibodies or exogenous TGFβ3 (50 and 100 ng/100µL concentrations) at the time of wounding resulted in a significant improvement in subsequent scarring.[13–15,20] Scarring is a continuous spectrum of phenotypes, with outcomes determined by the interaction of cells with the changing molecular and cellular microenvironments occurring during the process of wound healing and scarring. The results of these studies indicated that intradermal administration of TGFβ3 to approximated incisions reprograms the scarring response to result in a phenotype that more closely resembles fetal scar-free healing (**Fig. 3**).

The improvements in scarring achieved with TGFβ3 were accompanied by a histological improvement in skin architecture (**Fig. 4**). In normal skin, collagen has a characteristic basket weave

Table 1
Therapeutic approaches for the management of scarring

Surgery	Good surgical technique and design	
Peri-surgery	Prophylactic medicine promoting regeneration of normal skin, architecture (eg, avotermin [recombinant human TGFβ3])[a]	
Postsurgery	Silicone gel sheeting	Pressure garments
	Steroid injections	Hydrating creams and ointments
	Lasers	Other therapies: cryotherapy, radiotherapy, cytotoxics

[a] In clinical development (not yet approved).

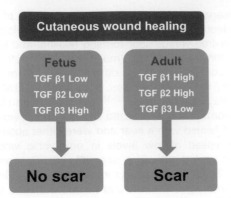

Fig. 2. Differential expression of TGFβ isoforms during healing of fetal and adult wounds.

arrangement with relatively thick bundles of collagen distributed in a loose and relatively random arrangement. By contrast, the arrangement of collagen in scarred skin demonstrates a markedly disrupted architecture with a less-random

arrangement. In a scar, the dermis contains densely packed, parallel bundles of collagen with reduced fibril diameter. Following intradermal administration of avotermin at the time of wounding, the architecture of collagen in the neodermis of the rat is improved compared with placebo and displays a more normal basket weave arrangement (see **Fig. 4**).

These experimental studies led to a preclinical program evaluating avotermin (recombinant human TGFβ3) as a therapeutic for prophylactic improvement of scarring. The scar improvement efficacy of avotermin was confirmed in a series of studies conducted in a rat model with full-thickness skin incisions. These showed that the efficacious doses of intradermal avotermin ranged between 50 to 500 ng/100μL per linear centimeter of wound margin. It also was confirmed in a clinically relevant pig model that intradermal administration of avotermin, at concentrations ranging 12 to 30 times higher than those predicted to be

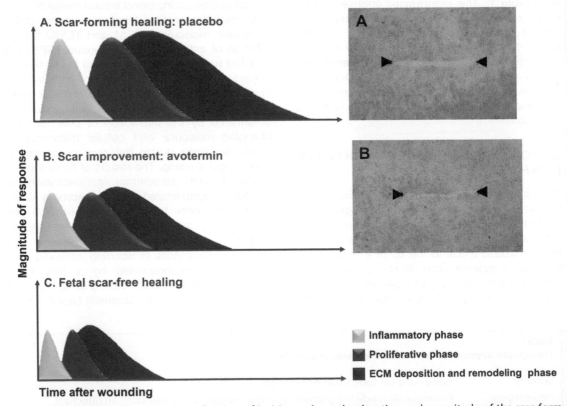

Fig. 3. Administration of avotermin at the time of incision reduces the duration and magnitude of the scar-forming healing response, with regenerated cutaneous tissue more closely resembling that of the normal surrounding skin. Full-thickness cutaneous incisional wounds in rats were treated around the time of wounding (once at the time of surgery and 24 hours later) with intradermal injections of placebo or avotermin and harvested 84 days later. The macroscopic appearance of scars at 70-days after wounding from wounds treated with (*A*) placebo and (*B*) avotermin at 50 ng/100 μL/linear cm of wound margin. *Arrowheads* indicate the ends of the original 1 cm wounds.

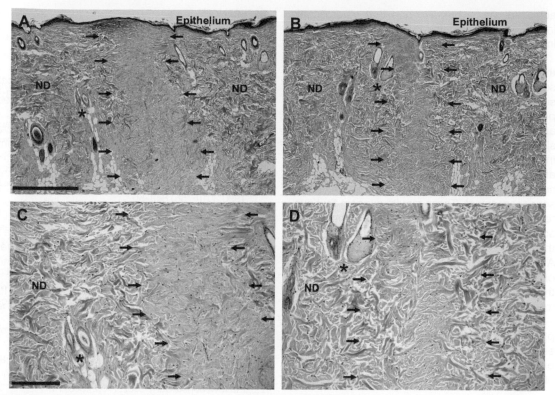

Fig. 4. Acute intradermal application of avotermin (TGFβ3) around the time of wounding to full-thickness skin incisions in the rat is associated with the regeneration of a dermal architecture that more closely resembles normal skin. The histological appearance of the repaired dermis/scars (indicated by *arrows*) at 70 days after wounding from wounds treated with placebo (*A, C*) and avotermin at 50 ng/100 μL/linear cm of wound margin (*B, D*) stained with Masson's Trichrome (collagen fibers stain green). Higher power images of the architecture of the repaired dermis show characteristic parallel bundles of fine collagen fibers in placebo-treated wounds that heal with scar formation (*D*), which is distinct to the basket weave organization of collagen bundles in the normal dermis (ND), while those in avotermin-treated wounds, which heal with reduced scarring, show a collagen organization more similar to normal dermis. Scale bars in (*A*) and (*C*) are 500 mm and 200 mm respectively; *indicates hair follicles.

efficacious in people, is tolerated well at the dosing site, does not affect wound healing or wound strength adversely, has low bioavailability, is cleared rapidly, and has no systemic toxicity (Laverty and colleagues manuscript submitted).

CLINICAL DEVELOPMENT OF AVOTERMIN FOR THE PROPHYLACTIC IMPROVEMENT OF SCARRING

The clinical development of avotermin as a prophylactic agent for improving scarring has progressed through a series of phase 1 and 2 human studies. These investigated the safety and efficacy of avotermin in terms of dose ranging and dosing frequency, with a view to defining the optimal dose and schedule. In all studies, avotermin was administered as an intradermal injection around the time of surgery. The phase 2 program

comprised a series of prospective, within-subject controlled, double-blind, placebo-controlled randomized clinical trials with predefined efficacy end points in human volunteers. These studies enabled well-controlled and robust proof-of-concept testing of the scar improvement efficacy and safety of avotermin in people.

To date, seven double-blind, placebo-controlled, randomized human phase 1/2 clinical trials have established that intradermal avotermin administered at doses of 50 to 500 ng/100μL per linear centimeter wound margin results in statistically significant improvements in scar appearance compared with placebo or standard care, with data showing that avotermin-treated scars more closely resemble surrounding normal skin (manuscripts submitted and in preparation). The studies have shown that short- and longer-term (to at least 12 months after wounding) improvements are achieved with avotermin, and that macroscopic improvements are underpinned by histological improvements in scar architecture.

Most recently, a phase 2 clinical trial has shown that avotermin is effective for improving unsightly scars, when administered following scar-revision surgery. Intradermal avotermin at 200 ng/100 µL per linear centimeter administered twice to each approximated wound margin following scar-revision surgery achieved a statistically significant improvement in scar appearance over 7-months after surgery compared with placebo, when assessed by a panel of lay volunteers trained in scar assessment. These results suggest that avotermin supplements good surgical technique for scar revision, resulting in less noticeable scars that more closely resemble the surrounding skin. A randomized, double-blind, placebo-controlled phase 3 study is being planned to further evaluate the clinical utility of avotermin administered following scar revision surgery.

More than 1000 people have been treated in the phase 1/2 clinical studies completed. These have established that avotermin has a favorable safety profile, which is characterized by a low incidence of site-specific adverse events.

SUMMARY

Patients and physicians are concerned about scarring resulting from routine elective and aesthetic procedures, and patients, in particular, value even small improvements in scarring. Translational research into the processes involved in scarring at the molecular, cellular, and tissue levels has facilitated the discovery and development of new biological approaches for improving scarring. Preclinical and clinical studies have provided evidence that avotermin (human recombinant TGFβ3) is the first in a new class of prophylactic medicines that may promote the regeneration of normal skin and improve scar appearance. Administered at the time of surgery, avotermin has potential to add to good surgical technique for the improvement of postoperative skin scarring.

ACKNOWLEDGEMENTS

The authors would like to thank Kathryn Quinn, Renovo, for help with preparation of the manuscript and Mark Ferguson, Nick Occleston, Andrew Kay, and John Hutchison for helpful comments and advice.

REFERENCES

1. Rumsey N, Clarke A, White P. Exploring the psychosocial concerns of outpatients with disfiguring conditions. J Wound Care 2003;12(7):247–52.
2. Bisson JI, Shepherd JP, Dhutia M. Psychological sequelae of facial trauma. J Trauma 1997;43(3):496–500.
3. Young VL, Hutchison J. Insights into patient and clinician concerns about scar appearance: semiquantitative structured surveys. Plast Reconstr Surg 2009, in press.
4. Shepherd JP, Qureshi R, Preston MS, et al. Psychological distress after assaults and accidents. BMJ 1990;301(6756):849–50.
5. Ferguson MW, O'Kane S. Scar-free healing: from embryonic mechanisms to adult therapeutic intervention. Philos Trans R Soc Lond B Biol Sci 2004;359(1445):839–50.
6. American Society of Plastic Surgeons. Plastic surgery growth in 2007. Available at: http://www.plasticsurgery.org/media/statistics/index.cfm. Accessed October 6, 2008.
7. Bayat A, McGrouther DA. Clinical management of skin scarring. Skinmed 2005;4(3):165–73.
8. Mustoe TA, Cooter RD, Gold MH, et al. International clinical recommendations on scar management. Plast Reconstr Surg 2002;110(2):560–71.
9. Reish RG, Eriksson E. Scars: a review of emerging and currently available therapies. Plast Reconstr Surg 2008;122(4):1068–78.
10. Reish RG, Eriksson E. Scar treatments: preclinical and clinical studies. J Am Coll Surg 2008;206(4):719–30.
11. Durani P, Bayat A. Levels of evidence for the treatment of keloid disease. J Plast Reconstr Aesthet Surg 2008;61(1):4–17.
12. Whitby DJ, Ferguson MW. Immunohistochemical localization of growth factors in fetal wound healing. Dev Biol 1991;147(1):207–15.
13. Shah M, Foreman DM, Ferguson MW. Control of scarring in adult wounds by neutralising antibody to transforming growth factor beta. Lancet 1992;339(8787):213–4.
14. Shah M, Foreman DM, Ferguson MWJ. Neutralisation of TGF-beta 1 and TGF-beta 2 or exogenous addition of TGF-beta 3 to cutaneous rat wounds reduces scarring. J Cell Sci 1995;108:985–1002.
15. Shah M, Foreman DM, Ferguson MW. Neutralising antibody to TGF-beta 1,2 reduces cutaneous scarring in adult rodents. J Cell Sci 1994;107(Pt 5):1137–57.
16. Bandyopadhyay B, Fan J, Guan S, et al. A traffic control role for TGFβ3: orchestrating dermal and epidermal cell motility during wound healing. J Cell Biol 2006;172(7):1093–105.

17. Chen W, Fu X, Ge S, et al. Ontogeny of expression of transforming growth factor-beta and its receptors and their possible relationship with scarless healing in human fetal skin. Wound Repair Regen 2005;13(1): 68–75.

18. O'Kane S, Ferguson MWJ. Transforming growth factor betas and wound healing. Int J Biochem Cell Biol 1997;29(1):63–78.

19. Occleston NL, Laverty HG, O'Kane S, et al. Prevention and reduction of scarring in the skin by transforming growth factor beta 3 (TGFβ3): from laboratory discovery to clinical pharmaceutical. J Biomater Sci Polym Ed 2008;7(3):1047–63.

20. Durani P, Occleston N, O'Kane S, et al. Avotermin: a novel antiscarring agent. Int J Low Extrem Wounds 2008;7(3):160–8.

Index

Note: Page numbers of article titles are in **boldface** type.

Clin Plastic Surg 36 (2009) 315–317
doi:10.1016/S0094-1298(09)00018-2
0094-1298/09/$ – see front matter © 2009 Elsevier Inc. All rights reserved.

Moving?

Make sure your subscription moves with you!

To notify us of your new address, find your **Clinics Account Number** (located on your mailing label above your name), and contact customer service at:

E-mail: elspcs@elsevier.com

800-654-2452 (subscribers in the U.S. & Canada)
314-453-7041 (subscribers outside of the U.S. & Canada)

Fax number: 314-523-5170

Elsevier Periodicals Customer Service
11830 Westline Industrial Drive
St. Louis, MO 63146

*To ensure uninterrupted delivery of your subscription, please notify us at least 4 weeks in advance of move.

Printed and bound by CPI Group (UK) Ltd, Croydon, CR0 4YY

03/10/2024

01040362-0003